From the experts at *Cooking Light*

THE 10 POUNDS OFF GLUTEN-FREE DIET

The Easy Way to Drop Inches in Just 28 Days

Oxmoor
House®

Mixed Berry Muffins, page 83

CONTENTS

WHO DOESN'T WANT TO SEE THE SCALE 10 POUNDS LIGHTER? This book will show you how to do just that while adhering to a gluten-free eating plan. In the following pages, you'll find a comprehensive introduction to the diet (complete with cutting-edge research) as well as 100 recipes from the healthy cooking experts at *Cooking Light*, four weeks of meal plans, and a do-anywhere fitness plan to help you tone up and slim down—safely, easily, and deliciously.

PART 1

GLUTEN-FREE
POWER

GLUTEN FREE AND YOUR HEALTH

GLUTEN HAS BEEN A BUZZ-WORD FOR THE LAST FEW YEARS. You probably know people who have gone gluten free and wondered what it might do for you. As a diet concept, going gluten free has been increasing by leaps and bounds. You can find gluten-free foods at most supermarkets, delis, and restaurants. There is even gluten-free beer, which is quite a trick when you consider the importance of gluten-containing barley to the beer-making process.

TIP

Helpful definitions
• *Celiac disease* is a genetic disorder in which gluten damages the lining of the small intestine, leading to a number of physical and neurological symptoms that vary from person to person. Gluten must be avoided for life.
• *Gluten sensitivity* (GS) and *gluten intolerance* (GI) are often used interchangeably. Individuals have trouble digesting gluten and don't feel well after eating it. While these conditions share some of the same symptoms of celiac disease, GI and GS patients have not shown damage to their small intestine.
• A *wheat allergy* causes an allergic reaction to wheat, but people with this allergy may be able to tolerate other grains, such as oats, rye, and barley, since the allergy is not in response to gluten.

Gluten is a combination of proteins found in wheat, barley, rye, and triticale (a wheat/rye hybrid). In bread making, gluten develops as the dough is kneaded, making it springier. For some people, the protein can cause severe difficulties with their digestive tract (more about that later). Others believe that they might have a sensitivity to gluten that could be causing them to gain weight or suffer achy joints and headaches, among other health problems.

Individuals with celiac disease, which is an immune response to gluten, have difficulty absorbing nutrients from certain foods and may end up *losing* weight, not gaining it. Those with gluten sensitivity, whose symptoms include diarrhea or abdominal pain, may also lose weight prior to restricting gluten from their diet, but others with gluten-related issues may still struggle with their weight. If you suspect you have celiac disease or a wheat allergy, you should speak to a medical professional to get the appropriate testing done before going on a gluten-free diet. (There is no diagnostic test to confirm gluten sensitivity or gluten intolerance.) It's more difficult to diagnose these issues if you give up gluten before being tested. If you test negative, you could eliminate gluten from your diet to see if your symptoms improve, which would imply a gluten sensitivity.

The Perfect Way to Lose 10 Pounds

When you set out to shed just a few pounds, the last thing you want to do is adopt a complex eating system. A huge advantage of going gluten free is that you don't have to weigh food, do elaborate planning for meals, or count calories or points. That may seem liberating—or possibly a little frightening, if you're accustomed to diets with rigid calorie- or points-counting rules.

By eliminating gluten, you won't have to count calories because you'll naturally avoid many of the foods that lead to weight gain. This diet encourages you to eat whole foods and avoid highly processed foods—including the gluten-free options—that are often high in calories, refined carbohydrates, fat, and added sugar. Eating the foods you're meant to consume will help you naturally feel full before you're at risk of overeating. Plus, you'll stay satisfied for much longer than when you eat the cheap, nutritionally unfulfilling foods so common in our modern diet. Although dieting experts set the pace of safe weight loss at 2 pounds per week, once you start your gluten-free diet, you may be surprised that you lose more than that in the first several weeks.

The Right Diet for Shedding Pounds

Look, you probably know that if you eat fewer calories than you burn through exercise and daily activity, you will lose weight. But one thing researchers have learned in the last decade is that there's nothing simple about how the calories you eat influence appetite. The biggest surprise was that low-fiber carbohydrates—think of white-flour bread and crackers, and low-fat, high-sugar treats—could actually *increase* hunger. These simple, easily digested carbohydrates break down more rapidly and cause a bigger increase in your blood sugar than carbohydrates that contain more fiber and take longer to digest. The sudden surge of glucose provokes a rise in insulin, the hormone your body relies on to process sugar. All that glucose either gets burned up for energy or shuttled off to places like your thighs and belly to be converted to long-term storage—in other words, fat.

The rapid peak and then plunge in blood sugar is a source of weight-gain troubles. As levels fall, your gut signals to your brain that energy supplies are running low, and just like that, you're hungry again or have less energy. The calories you consumed are responsible for making you want to eat more, and suddenly the calories in vs. calories out equation doesn't add up the way we always thought it did.

The solution is to add more lean protein (fish, lean cuts of meat, and nuts), high-fiber carbohydrates (brown rice, amaranth, millet, and certified gluten-free oats), and healthy fats to your diet. All these foods take longer to digest, resulting in a more gradual rise of blood sugar. You'll feel full longer and give yourself a chance to tip the scale in your favor.

Beginning a new plan will fill you with energy so you may be more active. Within a week or two you'll find that your face and shape are noticeably different when you gaze in the mirror!

Lose Belly Fat Faster

Incorporating more lean protein into your gluten-free diet has some other benefits. Carrying extra pounds around the midsection may be the most troubling aspect of being overweight. Research has found that too much fat in your belly is harder on organs, arteries, and the heart than fat you carry elsewhere, such as on your hips or thighs. According to new research, diets high in protein might help you target your spare tire.

At McMaster University in Ontario, researchers recruited 90 overweight and obese women and put them on a regular exercise schedule of walking and strength training. They also assigned them to one of three diets, featuring high, medium, and low amounts of protein. The researchers measured the volunteers' fat and muscle both at the beginning of the study and four months later, at the end. While all the women lost the same amount of weight on average, the big difference was in their levels of fat

> "When you feel better, there is a domino effect. I deal with stress better, sleep well, and no longer worry about what I'm going to eat."

Success Story:
Carmen

BEFORE

Age: **42**

Height: **5'2"**

Weight before: **143**

Weight after: **130**

Carmen searched for an answer to ongoing GI problems, trying multiple physicians who repeatedly told her, "It's all in your head." Finally, one physician listened to Carmen and tested her for gluten-related conditions. He recommended she follow a gluten-free eating plan. It worked so well that she lost 13 pounds and found relief from GI flare-ups. Her orthopedic physician was thrilled with the weight loss as well, due to Carmen's hip dysplasia, which is managed more effectively at a healthy weight. The weight loss also helped Carmen achieve the highest level of fitness in her employer's wellness program and earned her a substantial financial reward.

"I feel better and don't have to worry about GI problems like I did in the past. When you feel better, there is a domino effect. I deal with stress better, sleep well, and no longer worry about what I'm going to eat. It's really freed me to live without fear of what I eat."

Pounds lost: 13

AFTER

and muscle: 100 percent of the weight loss in the high-protein group was fat, especially around the midsection.

What's more, they added about a pound and half of muscle, while the low-protein group actually lost 1.5 pounds of muscle. "The preservation or even gain of muscle is very important for maintaining metabolic rate and preventing weight regain, which can be a major problem for many seeking to lose weight," says Andrea Josse, lead author of the study and a graduate student in the Department of Kinesiology at McMaster University.

How much protein did the women consume? The amounts weren't too daunting: They got about 30 percent of their calories from protein—about what you'd get on a gluten-free plan; most Americans typically get in the neighborhood of 15 to 20 percent.

TIP

Decide the best way for *you* to make a change. Some people like to remove all the off-limits food at once. Others thrive when they eliminate one food group at a time—start by getting rid of wheat, for example, then, a week or two later, processed sugars. Think about which approach sounds more appealing to you.

A study from Denmark is just the latest to underscore the importance of cutting back on carbohydrates in favor of lean, healthy protein. Nutrition researchers at the University of Copenhagen put 744 obese adults on several different diets that ranged from a traditional low-protein (13 percent of total calories) plan to one that got about 25 percent of its calories from protein. Each diet received a fairly liberal 25 to 30 percent of calories from fat.

After eight weeks, each group had lost an average of 24 pounds, although nearly 40 percent of the high-carb group dropped out, compared to just 25 percent of the high-protein group. But the true advantage to increasing protein became apparent six months later when the researchers followed up with the dieters. Those who had followed the high-carb plan had regained an average of roughly 4 pounds, while the high-protein group averaged less than 2 pounds of weight regain.

In addition to eating more healthy protein like turkey and fish, the successful dieters added quality, high-fiber carbohydrates such as brown rice, say the researchers. The advantage to high-fiber carbs is that they slow down digestion, allowing you to feel full longer. Protein also takes longer to digest—a diet composed of these foods will keep your gut busy, reducing hunger between meals.

The Benefits of a Gluten-Free Diet

Health is one of the biggest concerns—and reasons—dieters debate when adopting this plan. In fact, some researchers and diet experts still debate whether an approach that encourages protein and eliminates many carbohydrate-rich foods can really be safe. But rest assured that you can cut back on gluten for weeks or months and not worry about your health.

Obviously, a gluten-free diet offers great health benefits to those individuals diagnosed with celiac disease, gluten sensitivity, and wheat allergies; it's also sometimes recommended for children with autism. Celiac disease is a digestive disorder in which gluten damages the lining of the small intestine and reduces its ability to absorb vital nutrients. This condition is an autoimmune one rather than a food allergy, as gluten-containing food actually causes damage to the lining of the small intestine. This damage increases the risk of malnutrition because the small intestine can't effectively absorb nutrients. Common symptoms include diarrhea, constipation, gas, bloating, weight loss, nausea, vitamin deficiencies, and severe abdominal pain, but gluten can also cause further damage and additional symptoms in other areas of the body. The range and severity of symptoms varies greatly among individuals, and the level of gluten in certain foods affects each person differently. The only treatment is a lifelong gluten-free diet.

Persons with gluten sensitivity can exhibit a wide range of reactions, from digestive issues to headaches, balance problems, and many other

> **TIP**
>
> **When you're eliminating gluten, pick up the slack with more produce.** A smart thing to do when you start this plan is to make sure your house is stocked with plenty of healthy produce. Keep in-season fruit in bowls on your counters and dining table and in your fridge.

Recruit a partner.
Getting your spouse, friend, or family member to join you will help you get off to a good start. The two of you can share ideas and recipes, and keep each other on track through the tough times. One thing is for certain: Taking efforts to eliminate gluten from your diet *will* help you shed pounds. Essentially, you'll be eliminating a lot of the cheap carbohydrates that are directly related to weight gain. You'll also increase your protein intake, and there are a lot of good studies that suggest that eating high-quality, lean protein can help you slim down.

difficulties. And these symptoms may range from mild to severe. The only treatment for gluten sensitivity is avoidance of gluten. Individuals with allergies must avoid wheat proteins, which include gluten. Symptoms can include hives, nasal congestion, nausea, and anaphylaxis. The only treatment is avoidance of wheat products. Some physicians prescribe a diet free of gluten and casein (a milk protein) to improve behavior in children with autism. Not all autistic children respond to a gluten-free/casein-free diet (known as a GFCF diet), and it is typically used as a part of the overall treatment.

Lactose Intolerance

Some people who cannot eat gluten also experience lactose intolerance—gluten-induced damage to the intestines can decrease the ability to digest lactose. For the recipes in this book containing dairy products, you can make ingredient substitutions using dairy-free plain yogurts and cheeses, dairy-free buttery spreads in place of butter, and dairy-free beverages such as plain rice, soy, almond, coconut, or hemp milk in place of cow's milk. Please note that these products often have different textures and flavors compared to their dairy-containing counterparts, so you may need to experiment with the recipes to get the results you like.

Other Health Benefits

Weight loss alone can help reduce your risk of many chronic diseases, such as heart disease, diabetes, and several forms of cancer. By eating more healthy lean protein, gluten-free whole grains, and healthy fats, you'll go even further toward protecting yourself.

Healthy fats and proteins have surged to the forefront of good nutrition. We've come a long way from just 10 years ago, when government health experts and most major health organizations insisted that getting more than 30 percent of your calories from fat would blow you up like a balloon. Studies at Harvard revealed that people following low-fat diets lost less weight and were more likely to abandon their diets compared to people who followed regimens based on the Mediterranean diet, which contained as much as 40 percent of calories from fat (an amount that was once thought to be risky). A few years later, research on high-protein plans found that the higher amounts of fat in these diets didn't raise the risk of heart disease; in some studies, eating more fat actually lowered certain risk factors like cholesterol and artery inflammation.

Some newer studies even show that saturated fat may not be as bad as initially suspected. Certain foods that are higher in saturated fats, such as dark chocolate and eggs, have other healthy qualities like antioxidants, vitamins, and minerals that can enhance your diet.

One reason dieters benefit from adding healthy fat to their diets is that it tastes better, and it's more satisfying than simple carbohydrates. So go ahead and make more room in your weight-loss plan for avocados, eggs, olive oil, walnuts, oily fish like salmon, and lean cuts of beef. There's absolutely no reason why you can't eat well and still reach your goal weight.

WHY GOING GLUTEN FREE IS GOOD FOR YOU

THE ZONE. ATKINS. DUKAN. WEIGHT WATCHERS. ORNISH. All of these diets promote themselves as healthy ways to eat. Each plan comes with promises of dramatic weight loss. Yet they won't do you any good if you're gluten-sensitive. None of them takes into account the unique needs of the person who can't tolerate wheat, barley, rye, triticale, or anything that contains even a trace of gluten—a dizzying array of foods. Gluten is almost everywhere.

With the staggering increase in the number of people who respond poorly to gluten, more and more dieters are becoming frustrated with the alternatives and seeking out the only way of eating that will eliminate the source of their dietary troubles: They're going gluten free.

Just keep in mind that eating is supposed to make you feel good. When you sit down to a meal, the aftermath should not include gas, bloating, diarrhea, constipation, or nausea. Eating should make you feel energized, not headachy, fatigued, distracted, depressed, or awful.

For long-suffering gluten-sensitive people, this will come as a surprise. If you're in this group, you've no doubt spent a lifetime expecting and managing these unbearable symptoms. It's easy to assume that this is what life should be like: Eat, feel terrible, repeat. Gain weight, suffer achy joints, wrestle with migraines, and feel exhausted doing the most mundane activities.

The truth is that you don't have to live with pain and suffering. Change your diet, and those persistent, unpleasant symptoms will evaporate. You'll finally experience the gratification and satisfaction you should expect after replenishing your body.

Removing what is essentially a toxin from your diet will do wonders for your health. It's exactly that hope that drove you to purchase this book. What you may not realize is that there are other benefits to removing these grains from your diet, and altogether they add up to a far healthier way of living. Here are just a few.

Less Processed Food

One easy way to cut many sources of gluten out of your diet is to make your own meals at home rather than relying on packaged and prepared foods. As researchers probe the modern diet to find out why the way we eat causes us to gain weight, they repeatedly come back to one fundamental truth: Processed food, which is factory-produced; packed with salt, sugar, and artificial flavorings; stripped of vital nutrients; and often a source of gluten, equals disaster for the body. Despite the obvious downside of these foods, most diet plans allow you to use them in your daily meals. In fact, you'll find a lot of gluten-free processed foods. Some plans even produce their own processed meals for sale in your local grocery store.

The issue with these low-quality foodstuffs is that while they may temporarily fill you up, they actually leave your body starving for good nutrition. You feel hungry after a big meal because you're craving the missing vitamins and minerals, not to mention the phytonutrients, antioxidants, and other valuable disease-fighting substances in unprocessed foods.

Fast food falls into this category as well. You wouldn't believe how many chemicals and flavorings are pumped into the average burger from a fast food chain. The sodium and sugar content in the food you get is often astronomically high. This stuff has been tested and tinkered with in laboratories for decades until food scientists could arrive at a food that triggers extreme flavor sensations that keep the public wanting more. By cutting fast food out of your diet, you'll rediscover the true, satisfying, and pleasurable flavors of real food.

Plenty of Produce

Many popular diet plans promise quick and dramatic weight loss, but there are some that restrict fruits and vegetables, which are a key component of a healthy diet. An advantage to going gluten free over other diet plans is that it will force you to eat more produce.

Produce delivers plenty of valuable disease-fighting substances that can also help you lose weight. Dusky greens, vibrant oranges, and sweet tomatoes not only taste amazing, but they're also packed full of vital nutrients. Better yet, their calorie-to-nutrient ratio can't be beat. And this is the problem with many restrictive diet plans. Yes, you can lose weight, but only at the expense of a variety of fresh, colorful fruits and veggies. If you've ever tried one of these plans, you already know how wrong it feels to deny your body these valuable, tasty foods.

The Hidden Health Bonuses

One of the oddest aspects of going gluten free is that you're ridding your diet of foods that you've been taught are among the healthiest available. Wheat, barley, rye, and triticale contain vitamin E and plenty of fiber, and compose—in whole-grain form—a complete nutritional package. While giving up these grains may initially give you pause, there's research that suggests our digestive tracts aren't really set up to deal with these grains at all.

From an evolutionary perspective, farming practices are relatively new to humans. Our ancestors, who, after all, are the architects of our current digestive system, evolved eating primarily what they could scavenge from trees and bushes (fruits, vegetables, nuts, and seeds) and what they could hunt and kill (meat and fish). Research suggests that our digestive tract thrives while digesting these ancestral foods but can struggle when trying to process more recently developed agricultural products, such as—you guessed it—wheat, barley, rye, and triticale. And gluten seems to be the root of the trouble.

For those who have celiac disease or wheat allergy, the damage done to the gastrointestinal tract means many nutrients are not absorbed. Your ability to digest *all* foods, not just grains, can be compromised. In a world of easy access to cheap fast food, one of the side effects of malnutrition can be overeating. When the body is craving vital vitamins and minerals it's missing, it triggers the release of hormonal signals that stimulate hunger, researchers at the University of Chicago have found. Cleansing your diet of these gluten-containing grains can help ensure your body gleans the nutrients it craves from the foods you eat, and this can help you control your weight. But you may be surprised to learn that there are other benefits to cutting back on these grains.

- **Decreased hunger:** One of the challenges when dieting is recognizing when you're full. Some studies indicate that certain components in gluten can mess with the ability of leptin, a hormone that communicates between your stomach and your brain, to let your brain know you are full and to stop eating. Leptin resistance—when leptin isn't sending messages to your brain correctly—has been linked to an increased risk of becoming obese or overweight.
- **Fewer hormones:** One of the problems of our modern lifestyle is that we're exposed to too many hormones—especially xenoestrogens, which are found in pesticides, herbicides, and fungicides that factory farms use on crops, such as wheat, barley, rye, and triticale. These xenoestrogens can mimic the hormone estrogen, which may promote the retention of fat in the body.
- **Healthier thyroid:** To get soft, pillowy slices of bread, food makers rely on a chemical dough conditioner called potassium bromate. The problem is that this conditioner also happens to be an endocrine disruptor—in preliminary studies it has been shown to interrupt the flow of the body's natural hormones and has been linked to an increased risk of thyroid cancer. But long before it spurs tumor growth, the conditioner can slow down your thyroid. One of this gland's jobs is to regulate metabolism; as the gland's activity decreases, so does your metabolism. That equals fewer calories burned and more fat on your body.
- **Less starch:** Food scientists call a critical ingredient in bread—amylopectin A—the super starch. This sugar helps bread rise and become fluffy, but in your body it behaves just like white sugar: It dramatically raises blood sugar. That leads to inflammation and insulin resistance because your body must work extra hard to process all that sugar.

Why Gluten Free Is Nutritionally Healthy

A concern for people going gluten free is whether they'll get all the nutrients they need. The good news is that several studies have demonstrated that eating the full complement of gluten-free foods does in fact provide all the nutrients you need. Studies by Loren Cordain, Ph.D., one of the originators of the Paleo diet, which recommends avoiding all grains and is a loose way of going gluten free, has found that the diet can provide anywhere from double to 10 times the amount of your daily requirements for vitamins and minerals. You can rest assured that there's no reason to take supplements when you go gluten free.

Cutting out wheat, barley, rye, and triticale means you're also depriving yourself of some significant sources of fiber. Just remember that you'll be exploring a whole new world of gluten-free grains. From amaranth to teff, you'll discover that these whole grains, which are also rich in fiber, can make up for whatever you might be missing when you're eating gluten free. And don't forget that the extra fruit, vegetables, and seeds that are part of your regular eating repertoire also contain plenty of fiber.

What About All The Protein?

When you're gluten free, it's possible that more of your calories will come from protein. Don't be alarmed. In fact, you can take comfort in knowing that the protein content of your diet is trending upward. The latest research suggests that if you want to lose weight, adding more lean beef, poultry, and fish into your meals is exactly what you need. It may be exactly what you've been missing.

In 2009, researchers at the University of Illinois and Penn State University conducted a 12-month university study of 130 people looking to shed some pounds. Half of them followed a high-carbohydrate, low-fat, low-protein diet inspired by the USDA food pyramid. The rest followed a diet moderately high in protein, about what you'll get on the *10 Pounds Off Gluten-Free Diet*. The researchers taught the volunteers to shop and prepare meals based on the plan they were following, then tracked the dieters through an active four-month weight-loss phase and then for an additional eight months while the dieters attempted to maintain their loss.

After a year, the high-protein group had lost 23 percent more weight—and kept it off—than the low-fat dieters. It was a clear win for high-protein eating, but the news was even better than at first blush. When the researchers analyzed the volunteers' bodies, they discovered that the high-protein group had lost 22 percent more body fat during the four-month weight-loss phase than the low-fat group.

Even more remarkable, the high-protein group continued to shed body fat through the eight-month maintenance phase. At the end of 12 months, the high-protein dieters had lost 38 percent more body fat than the low-fat group. How could this happen? The researchers believe that the boost in filling, slow-to-digest protein helped control hunger and reduce snacking. The additional protein created an environment in the body that encouraged the growth of muscle; because muscles burn more calories than fat, the diet created a self-sustaining weight maintenance process, the researchers theorize.

The findings underline the true value of eating more protein: Yes, you'll lose more weight because you'll feel fuller than you would on a high-carbohydrate plan. But you'll also preferentially shed unhealthy and unsightly body fat while preserving your calorie-burning muscles. By the way, the other finding from the study was that, at year's end, more than half of the low-fat group had dropped out of the study, while two-thirds of the high-protein dieters were still going strong. The bottom line: Going gluten free will not only help heal your gut; it may be the quickest, most effective, and easiest way to drop weight.

THE NUTS AND BOLTS OF GOING GLUTEN FREE

DEPENDING ON YOUR LEVEL OF SENSITIVITY, the effects of exposure to even a little gluten can be severe. As a result, you'll need to use vigilance in avoiding foods that contain it. You probably already know it's in breads, pastas, crackers, and cereals made with wheat, barley, rye, or triticale. But thanks to gluten's texture and binding qualities, it also turns up in stocks, sauces, salad dressings, chips, spices, deli meats, fast food, and candy. You can even find it in beauty products.

To eliminate gluten from your life, you'll have to develop your detecting skills. You'll need to read labels closely and learn to watch for the ingredients that may contain gluten—it's usually in one of the ingredients, not listed on its own. You may even need to call the manufacturer to verify that a product is gluten free. Oats, for example, don't contain gluten, but they're often processed on the same equipment as gluten-containing grain and therefore can be cross-contaminated.

Don't despair, though: Numerous gluten-free products are available in stores and online—from baking mixes and flours to pizza doughs and pastas—and new products are added all the time. While many gluten-free products, like sauces and condiments, can be used interchangeably with their gluten-containing counterparts, some need to be handled differently. These include primarily products that would normally contain gluten (breads, pastas, baking mixes, desserts) but have been made with gluten-free ingredients. When cooking with such foods, be sure to reference the packages and use the cooking instructions specified for that product. Various brands of the same product can also act differently based on the mix of ingredients and the amounts of each ingredient they contain, so a procedure and cooking time that worked perfectly for quinoa pasta won't always work for rice pasta, and one pancake mix may have a different texture than another. Follow the package directions and our instructions in the recipes closely for the best results.

Of course, there's another way to avoid gluten: If you make the effort to prepare most of your food at home using fresh ingredients, you'll have the most control over what goes into your body. Fresh ingredients, like fresh produce, lean protein, and gluten-free whole grains, are healthier choices than packaged foods, even if they are gluten free. Once you've stocked your kitchen, you'll be able to prepare gluten-free meals without a worry.

On the following pages we'll guide you to the foods you can keep on hand to make delicious meals that are also gluten free. And in some cases, when you need to make substitutions, we'll explain how to make gluten free work for baking and other uses.

Foods You Can Eat

Although you might feel like you're entering a strange new world of strict limitations when you go gluten free, there are a surprising number of familiar foods still on the menu. The following foods can fit into your new way of eating with ease. Just remember: If you want to trust that these foods are gluten-free, you must buy them unseasoned, unprocessed, and unprepared—in their most natural state, in other words.

Beans	Meat
Dairy	Nuts and seeds
Eggs	Poultry
Fish	Shellfish
Fruits	Vegetables

Good Grains and Starches

There are numerous grains that don't contain gluten. And yes, it *is* possible to bake and still be gluten free. Below is a list of the safe grains.

Amaranth	Polenta
Arrowroot	Potato flour
Buckwheat	Potato starch
Corn	Potatoes
Cornstarch	Quinoa
Grits	Rice
Hominy	Sorghum
Millet	Tapioca
Montina™ (Indian ricegrass)	Teff
Oats*	

*Choose oats marked "certified gluten free" since there's a risk of cross-contamination.

Below you'll find a list of alternative flours you can experiment with to help create your favorite baked goods.

ALMOND MEAL FLOUR: Ground from whole, blanched almonds, this high-protein flour adds a superb texture and nutty flavor.
Shelf life: Store in an airtight container in refrigerator or freezer up to six months.
Best for: biscuits, pancakes, waffles, muffins, cookies, piecrusts, and cakes

AMARANTH FLOUR: This flour is made from amaranth seeds that have been ground into dense flour.
Shelf life: Store in an airtight container in refrigerator or freezer up to six months.
Best for: pancakes, crepes, muffins, breads, crackers, and cookies

ARROWROOT STARCH: This tasteless white flour derived from the base of the arrowroot plant is an excellent substitute for cornstarch in baked goods.
Shelf life: Store in an airtight container in a cool, dry place up to six months.
Best for: breads and biscuits

BROWN RICE FLOUR: This flour is a staple in gluten-free baking. It's dense with a grainy texture and nutty flavor and works best when blended with other gluten-free flours.
Shelf life: Store in an airtight container in refrigerator up to six months.
Best for: pancakes, waffles, crepes, piecrusts, biscuits, muffins, cookies, cakes, and pastries

BUCKWHEAT FLOUR: Despite its name, buckwheat flour doesn't contain any wheat. Rather, buckwheat is a grain-like seed that's ground into flour. It has an earthy, nutty flavor.

Shelf life: Store in an airtight container in refrigerator up to six months or in freezer up to one year.
Best for: breakfast cereals, breads, pancakes, and waffles

COCONUT FLOUR: Coconut flour is ground from dried, defatted coconut meat. It works best when combined with other gluten-free flours.
Shelf life: Store in an airtight container in refrigerator or freezer up to six months.
Best for: pancakes, cakes, muffins, and breads

CORN FLOUR: Corn flour is ground from whole corn kernels into a texture much finer than traditional cornmeal. Variations include masa harina, which is ground from white or yellow corn, and harinilla, which is ground blue corn.
Shelf life: Store in an airtight container in refrigerator up to six months or freezer up to one year.
Best for: breads, pizza crusts, muffins, pancakes, cakes, and tortillas

CORNMEAL: Ground from whole corn kernels into a gritty meal, cornmeal is much coarser than corn flour. It adds a sweet, nutty flavor to a variety of baked goods.
Shelf life: Store in an airtight container in a cool, dry place up to two months or in refrigerator up to six months.
Best for: breads, muffins, pizza crusts, and tortillas

CORNSTARCH: This is a flavorless, fine white powder that adds airiness to gluten-free baked goods. It works best when blended with other gluten-free flours.
Shelf life: Store in an airtight container in a cool, dry place up to two years.
Best for: pancakes, muffins, biscuits, breads, and cakes

FLAXSEED MEAL: Made from flaxseeds that have been ground into a dense flour, flaxseed meal works best when blended with other gluten-free flours.
Shelf life: Store in an airtight container in refrigerator up to six months or freezer up to one year.
Best for: pancakes, waffles, muffins, and breads

HAZELNUT FLOUR: This sweet, tawny, high-protein flour is made from finely ground hazelnuts.
Shelf life: Store in an airtight container in refrigerator up to six months.
Best for: breads, muffins, cookies, and cakes

MILLET FLOUR: This highly nutritious flour is ground from millet grains. It imparts a sweet and nutty flavor to baked goods and also gives them a crumbly texture.
Shelf life: Store in an airtight container in refrigerator up to six months.
Best for: breads and muffins

OAT FLOUR: Oat flour is made from very finely ground oats. It adds a robust taste and hearty texture to baked goods. To avoid cross-contamination, purchase oat flour that's certified gluten free.
Shelf life: Store in an airtight container in a cool, dry place up to three months or in refrigerator or freezer up to six months.
Best for: muffins, breads, cookies, and cakes

INGREDIENT TIP

BUCKWHEAT

BUCKWHEAT is a misleading term. It's not wheat but rather a naturally gluten-free seed. It's a whole grain, which carries many health benefits such as helping to reduce blood cholesterol levels, and is less starchy and higher in fiber than gluten-free corn or rice.

QUINOA FLOUR: Ground from seeds, quinoa flour is a nutritious, high-protein flour that has a slightly nutty flavor.
Shelf life: Store in an airtight container in refrigerator up to six months.
Best for: biscuits, muffins, cookies, breads, and cakes

SORGHUM FLOUR: Sorghum flour is ground from a high-protein, high-fiber cereal grain. It is heavy and should be blended with lighter, starchier flours.
Shelf life: Store in an airtight container up to three months, in refrigerator up to six months, or in freezer up to one year.
Best for: muffins, pancakes, biscuits, cookies, cakes, and breads

SWEET POTATO FLOUR: When added to baked goods, sweet potato flour helps them retain moisture while enhancing nutrition and adding richness.
Shelf life: Store in an airtight container in a cool, dry place up to one year.
Best for: pancakes, crepes, breads, and muffins

TAPIOCA FLOUR (STARCH): A light, powdery, tasteless flour, tapioca flour adds body and chewy texture to baked goods. It works best when combined with other gluten-free flours.
Shelf life: Store in an airtight container in a cool, dry place up to two years.
Best for: pancakes, muffins, biscuits, cookies, cakes, and breads

TEFF FLOUR: This finely textured flour is milled from a grain named teff.
Shelf life: Store in an airtight container in refrigerator up to six months.
Best for: pancakes, muffins, breads, and tortillas

WHITE RICE FLOUR: This flour is derived from white rice that has been ground into a light, powdery flour. It is a gluten-free baking staple. Use it interchangeably with brown rice flour.

Shelf life: Store in an airtight container in a cool, dry place up to one year.

Best for: pancakes, waffles, crepes, piecrusts, biscuits, muffins, cookies, brownies, cakes, and pastries

The "Maybe" Foods

These foods may be made with or without gluten, so it is important to read labels to find a safe version. By law, companies have to list wheat on the label if it is found in any ingredient, but you'll still want to double-check. For more information on where gluten may hide, see "Decoding Food Labels" on page 38.

- Baked goods like bread, breadcrumbs, cakes, cookies, croutons, muffins, and piecrusts
- Beer
- Bouillon
- Breading and coating mixes
- Broth (all varieties)
- Candy
- Cereal
- Coated popcorn and chips
- Corn tortillas
- Crackers
- Energy bars
- Fast food
- Flavored alcoholic drinks
- Flavored or coated nuts and seeds
- Flavored teas
- Gravies, marinades, and sauces

Hoisin sauce

Licorice

Ice cream

Imitation seafood

Marinades

Multigrain rice and corn cakes

Oats (look for gluten-free oats)

Pastas

Pepperoni

Prepackaged convenience foods

Prepared icings and frostings

Prepared salsas

Processed foods

Processed meats (hot dogs, lunchmeat, and sausage)

Roasted nuts

Rotisserie chicken

Salad dressings

Sauces and gravies

Seasoned rice mixes

Seasoning mixes

Soups

Soy sauce

Spices (if there is no ingredient list on the label, then it contains only the pure spice)

Teriyaki sauce

Vegetables packaged with sauces

Worcestershire sauce

Yogurt (with granola)

INGREDIENT TIP

RICE

RICE can become an easy fallback when you're going gluten free. You'll find it's used to make gluten-free pasta, baked goods, and cereals. But Consumer Reports found small but measurable amounts of arsenic in most rice products, and the organization warns against relying too heavily on rice-based substitutes.

Decoding Food Labels

Reading food labels is a must. Sometimes, the distinctions between gluten-free and gluten-containing foods aren't obvious until you read the label. Food companies manufacture their products differently, and the ingredients often vary from brand to brand. So it's vital to learn the names of ingredients that could cause concern if you see them on food labels. With practice, patience, and time, label reading will become second nature.

BARLEY: Barley appears on labels as malt, malt extract, malt flavoring, malt syrup, malt vinegar, barley malt flavoring, barley malt syrup, and brown rice syrup (which may be made with barley enzymes). All of these terms indicate the presence of gluten, and the item should be avoided.

CARAMEL COLOR: This ingredient, when manufactured in North America, is produced from corn and is gluten free.

HYDROLYZED VEGETABLE PROTEIN: This term is not used on a label. Instead, the label must specify the vegetable or grain, such as "hydrolyzed wheat protein," which is not gluten free, or "hydrolyzed soy protein," which is gluten free.

MALTODEXTRIN: This ingredient is made from corn, potato, or rice and should not be confused with the barley-containing ingredients known as malt or malt flavoring. If wheat was used, the label would have to say "wheat maltodextrin," "maltodextrin (wheat)," "dextrates," and "dextri-maltose." The term "dextrin" is rarely used on food labels.

MODIFIED FOOD STARCH: This ingredient can be made from wheat, but the label must say "wheat."

WHEAT STARCH: The starch is used as a binder and thickening agent in foods. If it is used as an ingredient, the label must say "wheat."

> "I had no idea how life-changing it would be. It went beyond eating food. My body felt better."

Success Story:
Dorothy

Dorothy suffered from high blood pressure, internal inflammation, GI issues, swollen feet and ankles, and very low energy. Additionally, she was overweight. She never thought she could stick to a diet. When invited to participate in a 6-month gluten-free challenge, she decided to give it a try.

Focusing on eating healthier and accepting herself, Dorothy began to feel healthier and more confident. Her sweet tooth subsided and her hunger cravings decreased. Her blood pressure dropped and her swollen feet and ankles returned to normal. She learned to cook and planned her meals and snacks throughout her day. Most importantly, she had a support group and blogged about her experience. Dorothy saw the pounds shed and learned to love her body. "I had no idea how life-changing it would be. It went beyond eating food. My body felt better."

BEFORE

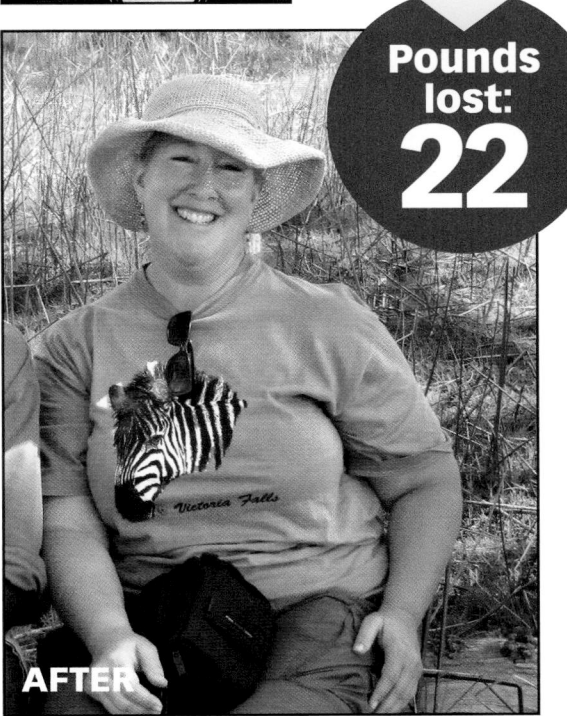

AFTER

Age: **52**

Height: **5'6"**

Weight before:
250

Weight after:
228

Pounds lost:
22

Foods to Avoid

The primary grains you need to avoid are wheat, barley, rye, triticale (a hybrid grain), and possibly oats (due to cross-contamination). But those are the primary forms of gluten. It can also turn up in other forms in foods, so refer to the following list when in doubt. Whether it's the primary ingredient or way down the list, the appearance of one of these items in the ingredients indicates that the food contains gluten.

Barley

Barley malt

Bran (oat, wheat)

Brewer's yeast

Bulgur

Cooking spray for baking (may contain wheat flour)

Couscous

Durum

Einkorn

Emmer

Farina

Farro

Flour containing wheat, barley, or rye or any of their derivatives

Graham flour

Hydrolyzed wheat protein

Kamut/khorasan wheat

Malted milk

Malt flavorings

Malt vinegar

Matzo

Meat, poultry, seafood, or vegetables that are breaded, floured, served with a sauce made from wheat, or marinated in a wheat-based sauce such as soy or teriyaki

Rye

Seitan

Semolina

Spelt

Triticale

Wheat

Wheat germ

Wheat starch

Wheatberries

Although there isn't much of a gluten concern with soda and diet soda, you'll still want to limit or eliminate your intake. Soda of course is loaded with sugar and no friend to weight-loss efforts. While diet soda and artificial sweeteners might seem harmless and a good alternative, they're not. Any savings they offer are illusory.

When Harvard researchers tracked people who primarily drank artificially sweetened beverages, they discovered that the diet soda drinkers gained more weight than people who drank regular soda (though both groups put on pounds). Back in the lab, the researchers discovered that when rats are given artificial sweeteners they actually eat more food than rats that get real sugar, possibly because calorie sensors in the gut and brain expect to gain energy from such a sweet taste. When the calories fail to turn up, these sensors prompted the rats to overeat to compensate.

The saccharin taste of these artificial sweeteners—which taste as much as a hundred times sweeter than sugar—presents another problem, say experts. We're training our taste buds to expect extreme flavors, and simple, good, sweet food like fruit pales in comparison. We end up shunning it in favor of the sensationally sweet foods.

Cut out the diet soda—and the regular soda. You'll miss them initially, but you can replace the drink with seltzer sweetened with a squeeze of lemon or lime. Within a week or two your taste buds will have recalibrated themselves, and you'll get more pleasure from a truly healthy (and weight-loss–friendly) diet.

PUTTING YOUR GLUTEN-FREE DIET INTO ACTION

NOW THAT YOU KNOW what you can and can't eat on your diet, it's time to clear out your kitchen. The easiest way to do this is if your entire household is going gluten free—then you can just donate or toss all the offending foods. However, it's unlikely this will be possible unless you live alone or with one other person.

If you're the only person making the gluten-free leap, try designating certain areas of your pantry, freezer, food shelves, and refrigerator as gluten-free zones.

TIP

What about alcohol?
You'll be happy to hear that most forms are okay. Beer is definitely a no-no (unless it's labeled gluten free), but wine, whiskey, gin, vodka, brandy, rum, and tequila are all gluten free!

Now take a hard look at the food in your house. This will be good practice for future shopping trips. Analyze the ingredient labels for signs of wheat, barley, and rye. Refer back to the list of possible pseudonyms for gluten ingredients on page 38. Check the cereal boxes, the boxes of "just add water" food products like macaroni and cheese, and canned soups.

Finding the primary offenders is easy: You can toss the bread and bagels; white and wheat flour; barley; bran; bulgur; malt vinegar; breaded meat, poultry, or fish; and the wheat germ as well as the crackers and cookies. And while you're at it, clear out the sodas and beer. If the food is unopened, you might be able to donate it. The rest a neighbor or relative might be open to taking.

GLUTEN-FREE SPICES

Once you've cleared the shelves, take a look at Chapter 6 on page 62 for a shopping list of gluten-free basics that you'll want to stock your cabinets with. One area you'll want to be sure is complete is your spice rack. Now that you'll be preparing more of your meals from scratch, spices are your ally. As long as there's only one ingredient on the label of the spice jar, it should be gluten free—but beware that some mixes may contain gluten. Here's a list of spices to keep on hand:

Bay leaves	Coriander	Mint
Black pepper	Crushed red pepper flakes	Oregano
Cayenne pepper	Cumin	Paprika
Cinnamon	Garlic powder	Rosemary
Cloves	Ginger	Salt
Cocoa	Ground mustard	Thyme

You may want to consider planting an herb garden as well, which allows you to have fresh herbs on hand at all times without having to run out to the grocery store. You can even grow herbs indoors with new kits on the market, and there's nothing like fresh basil, cilantro, rosemary, and thyme to liven up a dish.

Gluten-Free Tools

Here's a list of the tools and equipment you might need to create delicious gluten-free meals at home. A note on kitchen safety: If you also prepare foods that contain gluten in your kitchen, preventing cross-contamination is key. You'll need to thoroughly clean dishes, counters, cooking surfaces, and kitchen utensils and appliances after any of them have come into contact with foods containing gluten. (In a perfect world, separate appliances and small wares, such as cutting boards and flour sifters, would be best.) You probably have plenty of kitchen utensils and appliances on hand, but peruse this list to see if you're missing anything. These items aren't essential, but they will make preparing meals for your new eating plan much simpler.

KITCHEN SCALE Because each person scoops flour into a measuring cup differently, a kitchen scale is ideal because it allows for accurate measurements every time. A digital scale is the easiest to use, but a top-loading or hanging scale will also work.

LIQUID MEASURING CUPS Liquid measuring cups are usually made of glass, plastic, or stainless steel and are used to measure ingredients such as water, juices, milks, oils, and honey.

DRY MEASURING CUPS Dry measuring cups are usually made of plastic or stainless steel and are used to measure ingredients like flour, sugar, dried fruits, and nuts.

MEASURING SPOONS Measuring spoons are usually made of plastic, metal, or porcelain. They're used to measure smaller amounts of ingredients, such as spices, herbs, sugar, vanilla extract, baking soda, baking powder, xanthan gum, and yeast.

GRATER AND ZESTER These two essential pieces of equipment come in handy for grating a variety of ingredients like cheese, carrots, and zucchini. They are also needed to achieve the right texture, weight, and consistency when grating nutmeg or citrus rinds, which add flavor to baked goods.

HIGH-QUALITY KNIVES A sharp knife is a blessing in the kitchen. It turns a prep job from a chore to a pleasure. And the sharper the better: Dull knives are far more likely to slip and slice your finger than sharp ones. (So consider a high-quality sharpener to help maintain your knives' edges.)

SPIRALIZER This device can do wonderful things with vegetables to help them fill in for the grain foods you may be missing. You can turn squash, carrots, and other firm veggies into noodles for a pasta substitute, for noodles in a soup, or for an interesting textured filling in a lettuce wrap.

DIGITAL THERMOMETER When you'll be preparing lots of meat, this is an invaluable tool. The digital versions can give you a much faster read. Some include the option of leaving the sensor in the meat as it cooks in the oven or on the grill while the readout monitor sits on the counter so you know exactly when your meat is at the proper temperature.

EGG POACHERS Eggs are an excellent source of nutrition for gluten-free eaters. You may tire of fried eggs, scrambled eggs, and hard-cooked eggs, which is why having egg poachers on hand can help you keep your breakfasts feeling fresh. You can get silicone cups that float in boiling water, allowing you to poach eggs to perfection. Mix them with some quick-braised greens for a healthy start to your day.

8-INCH CAST-IRON SKILLET You'll find this skillet is perfect for whipping up a quick gluten-free breakfast, such as eggs and uncured ham. These pans typically come preseasoned, so all you have to do is be sure to keep it in shape. Use vegetable oil, canola oil, olive oil, or butter when you cook; rinse the skillet—no soap!—right after you finish and use a dishwashing brush to knock off the food scraps. Thoroughly dry the pan and smear a little of your cooking oil all over the top and bottom. Keep the skillet in a dry place that's handy. Food simply tastes better when made in these pans, and the care is so simple you'll wonder why you ever bothered with so-called nonstick cookware!

10- OR 12-INCH CAST-IRON SKILLET This larger skillet will be your go-to pan for cooking most of your dinner meals, whether it's searing steaks, crisping roasts that you'll finish in the oven (the great advantage of these pans is they can easily go from the stove top to the oven and back again), or whipping up stir-fries. Unlike most cookware, these hardy pans improve with age; their seasoning adds flavor to everything you cook. If you want to keep things simple, opt for this larger pan. You can use it to prepare smaller meals and breakfasts, too.

BAKING SHEETS Roasting vegetables like cauliflower, asparagus, and broccoli with olive oil, garlic, and pepper turns them into gourmet delights. Kale chips can stand in for any grain alternative. But to pull these dishes off with ease and panache, you'll need a good supply of baking sheets. Keep your cleanup quick and easy by lining the sheets with aluminum foil or parchment paper before baking.

TIP

Keep your kitchen safe. Cross-contamination with gluten can occur in food-processing plants—but it can also happen in your kitchen. If you're the only one going gluten free in your home, you'll want to keep duplicates of jarred foods that everyone eats, like peanut butter, and label the one that's yours. Otherwise, the knife used to spread peanut butter on bread will transfer small amounts of gluten to the jar.

SEPARATE CUTTING BOARDS If you prepare foods that contain gluten, it would be smart to purchase a cutting board specifically for prepping gluten-free ingredients. Cutting boards made of wood or bamboo have porous surfaces, which are hard to clean and have nooks and crannies where gluten can adhere.

STOCKPOT If you aren't making your own stock, now's the time to start. The store-bought stuff can be high in sodium and usually contains gluten. Drop a leftover chicken carcass or beef bones, roughly chopped onions, celery, carrots, and your choice of spices into a stockpot full of water, and let it simmer for an hour or so—you'll have the best stock you've ever had. Choose a big pot—20 quarts isn't too big. (You can always freeze your left-over stock.) If you don't have time to make your own, be sure to purchase reduced-sodium varieties of store-bought stock or broth.

MIXERS The three most popular baking mixers include the stand mixer, hand mixer, and immersion blender (also called a stick mixer). Electric mixers are designed to do the work for you and ensure that all the ingredients get mixed evenly and uniformly. They also have different speeds that allow you to whip delicate ingredients such as egg whites or thick ingredients such as brownie batter or marshmallows. A hand mixer or immersion blender is ideal for smaller jobs that don't involve mixing heavy batters or doughs.

FOOD PROCESSOR The food processor is a must-have, multitasking tool vital for every kitchen. It slices, chops, shreds, purees, grinds, and mixes a variety of ingredients—it is the most versatile piece of equipment in the kitchen and can be a huge time-saver when prepping ingredients.

BLENDER A blender is used to mix, blend, or emulsify food. It is great for pureeing fruit for pie fillings or toppings or blending smoothies; bean dips; or batters for pancakes, crepes, or waffles.

IMMERSION BLENDER This will come in handy morning, noon, and night. You can use it to easily puree soups or mix sauces and salad dressings.

SLOW COOKER The simplest way to save yourself time at the end of the day is to make dinner in the morning. Throw a bunch of fresh ingredients into your cooker along with broth and some bay leaves before you leave for work. Voilà: At the end of the day your dinner is ready and the house will smell wonderful.

GOOD STORAGE CONTAINERS Prepare double or triple batches of your favorite meals and freeze the leftovers in high-quality, freezer-durable containers. That's one or more meals you won't have to prepare down the road!

TAKE THE GLUTEN-FREE DIET CHALLENGE

RE YOU READY TO DIVE IN? Your kitchen is prepared, you have the food you need, and more importantly, you've eliminated the foods you need to avoid. Now it's time to take the challenge. On the following pages there are four weeks of food plans that will help you lose at least the 10 pounds you want to drop and control any symptoms you might be having. You'll also feel better, especially if you add the exercise component from Chapter 12.

WEEK 1

	BREAKFAST	LUNCH	DINNER
MONDAY	**Mixed Berry Muffins** (pg. 83)	**Spicy-Sweet Chicken Lettuce Cups** (pg. 100)	**Salsa Flounder** (pg. 108)
TUESDAY	**Peppery Potato Omelet** (pg. 69)	**Portobello and Black Bean Quesadillas** (pg. 103)	**Cast-Iron Burgers** (pg. 118)
WEDNESDAY	**Sunflower Granola** (pg. 75)	**Pork Wraps with Fresh Tomatillo Salsa** (pg. 98)	**Citrus-Herb Chicken** (pg. 124)
THURSDAY	**Mexican Chorizo Hash** (pg. 73)	**Broccoli-Cheese Soup** (pg. 104)	**Roasted Pork Tenderloin Tacos** (pg. 119)
FRIDAY	**Quinoa with Strawberries and Buttermilk** (pg. 77)	**Warm Brown Rice and Chickpea Salad with Cherries and Goat Cheese** (pg. 92)	**Five-Bean Chili** (pg. 135)
SATURDAY	**Mushroom Frittata** (pg. 70)	**Salmon Salad on Arugula** (pg. 89)	**Three-Cheese Baked Penne** (pg. 140)
SUNDAY	**Oatmeal Pancakes** (pg. 80)	**Blueberry Chicken Salad** (pg. 94)	**Vegetarian Lasagna** (pg. 139)

WEEK 2

	BREAKFAST	LUNCH	DINNER
MONDAY	Breakfast Quinoa (pg. 79)	Tuna-Pecan Salad Sandwiches (pg. 94)	Greek-Style Chicken Breasts (pg. 129)
TUESDAY	Mexican Chorizo Hash (pg. 73)	Roasted Carrot, Chicken, and Grape Quinoa Bowl (pg. 93)	Pasta Carbonara Florentine (pg. 143)
WEDNESDAY	Savory Buckwheat with Tomato, Cheddar, and Bacon (pg. 77)	Banh Mi–Style Roast Beef Sandwiches (pg. 97)	Sausage Pizza (pg. 138)
THURSDAY	Vanilla Amaranth with Peach Compote (pg. 76)	Chicken-Olive Quesadillas (pg. 102)	Pork Tenderloin and Cannellini Beans (pg. 121)
FRIDAY	Pecan-Oatmeal Waffles (pg. 82)	Spicy Steak Lettuce Wraps (pg. 95)	Chicken with Turnips and Pomegranate Sauce (pg. 126)
SATURDAY	Zucchini and Red Pepper Frittata (pg. 71)	Black Bean Soup (pg. 105)	Cedar Plank Salmon with Tomato Salsa (pg. 110)
SUNDAY	Cheesy Hash Brown Casserole (pg. 74)	Spicy Chicken Sandwiches (pg. 99)	Tomato-Basil Pasta with Asiago (pg. 141)

WEEK 3

	BREAKFAST	LUNCH	DINNER
MONDAY	**Pumpkinseed-Almond Granola** (pg. 75)	**Portobello and Black Bean Quesadillas** (pg. 103)	**Shredded Chicken Tacos with Tomatoes and Grilled Corn** (pg. 127)
TUESDAY	**Mexican Chorizo Hash** (pg. 73)	**Banh Mi–Style Roast Beef Sandwiches** (pg. 97)	**Tilapia Veracruz** (pg. 113)
WEDNESDAY	**Quinoa with Strawberries and Buttermilk** (pg. 77)	**Broccoli-Cheese Soup** (pg. 104)	**Slow-Cooker Brisket** (pg. 117)
THURSDAY	**Peppery Potato Omelet** (pg. 69)	**Pork Wraps with Fresh Tomatillo Salsa** (pg. 98)	**Saffron Rice with Tilapia and Shrimp** (pg. 111)
FRIDAY	**Blueberry-Almond Oatmeal Pancakes** (pg. 81)	**Spicy-Sweet Chicken Lettuce Cups** (pg. 100)	**Stuffed Poblanos** (pg. 137)
SATURDAY	**Breakfast Quinoa** (pg. 79)	**Roasted Carrot, Chicken, and Grape Quinoa Bowl** (pg. 93)	**Pork Tenderloin with Roasted Cherries and Shallots** (pg. 123)
SUNDAY	**Zucchini and Red Pepper Frittata** (pg. 71)	**Spicy Bean and Quinoa Salad with "Mole" Vinaigrette** (pg. 90)	**Braised Chicken with Honey-Lemon Leeks** (pg. 131)

WEEK 4

	BREAKFAST	LUNCH	DINNER
MONDAY	Cinnamon, Apple, and Oat Scones (pg. 84)	Blueberry Chicken Salad (pg. 94)	Seared Scallops with Snap Peas and Pancetta (pg. 115)
TUESDAY	Savory Buckwheat with Tomato, Cheddar, and Bacon (pg. 77)	Tuna-Pecan Salad Sandwiches (pg. 94)	Pasta with Roasted Red Pepper and Cream Sauce (pg. 142)
WEDNESDAY	Sunflower Granola (pg. 75)	Warm Brown Rice and Chickpea Salad with Cherries and Goat Cheese (pg. 92)	Chicken Verde Enchiladas (pg. 130)
THURSDAY	Mushroom Frittata (pg. 70)	Black Bean Soup (pg. 105)	Grilled Chicken Thighs with Cilantro-Mint Chutney (pg. 132)
FRIDAY	Mixed Berry Muffins (pg. 83)	Salmon Salad on Arugula (pg. 89)	Sautéed Tilapia Tacos with Grilled Peppers and Onion (pg. 114)
SATURDAY	Vanilla Amaranth with Peach Compote (pg. 76)	Chicken-Olive Quesadillas (pg. 102)	Dijon-Herb Chicken Thighs (pg. 134)
SUNDAY	Cheesy Hash Brown Casserole (pg. 74)	Spicy Steak Lettuce Wraps (pg. 95)	Asian Rice with Shrimp and Snow Peas (pg. 116)

Snacks

There are recipes for snacks (check out Edamame Crunch, pg. 150, Lemon-Parmesan Popcorn, pg. 151, and Roasted Garlic and Chive Dip, pg. 146), but for the most part, you'll want to experiment to find the snacks that work best in terms of filling you up and satisfying your cravings. Here are some other ideas you can experiment with:

Fresh fruit

Dried fruit

Raw vegetables

Guacamole

Hummus

Peanut butter

Gluten-free crackers

Gluten-free energy bars

Gluten-free cereal

Gluten-free tortilla chips

Nuts or seeds

Olives

Hard-cooked egg

String cheese

Greek yogurt

TIP

Go with what works. If you find a breakfast that works for your taste buds, time, and budget, feel free to stick with that. Same with lunch, although for dinner and snacks, you may want to try the suggestions in the plan so that you'll have a chance to experience different flavors and preparations.

Dessert

Pleasing your sweet tooth is easier than you might think when you're going gluten free. You'll find plenty of dessert options in Chapter 11 (pg. 164). One tip to remember is that you can use arrowroot flour to thicken dessert sauces (and regular sauces as well), though you'll want to use cornstarch if you're making a dairy-based sauce. When you don't have time to prepare a special dessert, look for gluten-free dark chocolate—stick to a square at a time to satisfy your sweets craving.

Eating Out Gluten Free

One of the easy ways to run into trouble when trying to stay gluten free is eating out. You may have noticed, though, that more and more restaurants are offering gluten-free entrées. However, if you're really sensitive, you'll have to verify that the food is prepared with separate pans and utensils to avoid cross-contamination. The following tips can help you navigate most menus and restaurants with ease.

- **Check out the menu online before you go.** With a little planning you can figure out where you'll eat and what you'll have before you leave the house. If you find that your destination offers gluten-free options, give the restaurant a call (just not during mealtime rush!) and query the staff about how the food is prepared.

- **Get to know your server/chef.** If you're eating out near your place of work, you probably have two or three places you go regularly. Don't hesitate to ask questions about how the food is prepared to make sure it conforms to your new diet.

- **Let the waitstaff know that you're gluten sensitive.** Most restaurants are ready to accommodate people who are gluten intolerant. If the staff seems unclear what that means, briefly explain which ingredients are off-limits for you.

- **Be flexible.** You might find that the restaurant is out of the dish you planned to order or that the staff can't satisfactorily answer your questions. Pack some gluten-free snacks just in case. You could also order a plate of fresh vegetables to nosh on while your companions eat.

TIP

Ask your waiter. It's okay to ask the waitstaff detailed questions about how food is prepared. Here are a few sample questions to tease out information:

- Are the French fries coated with flour?
- Are artificial bacon bits or other meat substitutes used on potato skins and salads?
- Does the salad dressing contain wheat or flour?
- Does the soup contain flour or barley?

Visit celiac.org for even more eating-out tips.

Eating Gluten Free on the Run

While preparing a beautiful meal and cooking more at home are the easiest ways to stay gluten free, the pressures of modern life often get in the way. Here are some ideas for quick breakfasts and lunches.

HARD-COOKED EGGS This is a simple, nutritious, and fast gluten-free breakfast. Pair it with some fresh fruit or kale chips, and you can start your day with a solid blast of nutrients and protein.

SMOOTHIE Throw some Greek yogurt, frozen berries, pineapple, mango, and ice into a blender for a smoothie that you can drink on your way to work and that will get you through your morning.

BARS AND MUFFINS You can find gluten-free breakfast muffins and energy bars at your local grocer. You can also make your own (so you can control the sugar). Check out the Mixed Berry Muffins (pg. 83), Cinnamon, Apple, and Oat Scones (pg. 84), Almond-Date Bars (pg. 175), and Maple-Pecan Bars (pg. 176).

TRAIL MIX Keep a plastic container full of your favorite roasted, unsalted nuts and dried fruit. Throw in some coconut flakes for variety.

BELL PEPPER OR CABBAGE SANDWICHES Slice bell pepper into wide, flat slabs, or peel off and wash sturdy, broad cabbage leaves to make sandwiches with sliced turkey, pitted olives, and the greens of your choice.

VEGGIES AND DIP Bring pieces of carrot, celery, broccoli, and cauliflower to dip in nut butter, hummus, or guacamole.

Traveling Gluten Free

When you're on the road, avoiding gluten can get a lot more difficult. One easy way to cover yourself is to pack a lot of snacks—they'll get you through situations where finding a gluten-free option may be tough. Here are some other tricks to keep in mind.

- **Find a gluten-free-friendly restaurant first.** If you can get a good breakfast to start your day, your battle is well on the way to being won.

- **Research local health/natural food stores.** If you don't want to waste time scanning grocery store shelves, you can get what you need here. The staff in these stores will be able to steer you to options and are more likely to be understanding and helpful about your sensitivity than the average chain grocery clerk.

- **Know your cuisines.** Mexican food can be gluten-free-friendly if you stick to the rice- or corn-based dishes. Watch out for the chips, flour tortillas, and anything that comes out of the deep fryer (no doubt the oil will also be used for gluten products). Thai cuisine is another great choice since the dishes typically rely on fish sauce (rather than the ubiquitous soy in Japanese and Chinese cuisines).

- **Pack plenty of options.** Let's face it, traveling adds plenty of challenges to remaining gluten free. So bring along a mini-pantry that can get you through the lean times, including bars, cereal, cookies, crackers, dried fruit, and nuts—pack as much as you can carry.

TIP

Cross-contamination concerns. When you're eating out, you should also ask your server about cross-contamination issues, like if there is a separate prep space for gluten-free foods, if separate utensils are used, and if they have a dedicated fryer (or change the frying oil) for gluten-free foods.

PART 2

100 GLUTEN-FREE RECIPES

YOU MAY BE GOING GLUTEN FREE, but eating good food is still vitally important. Gluten free doesn't mean flavor free, so you'll find all of your favorite foods—from burgers and pastas to muffins and cakes—in these recipe pages. A crucial step in staying gluten free will be keeping your pantry well stocked with gluten-free food. This will allow you to prepare any number of tasty meals at a moment's notice. All it takes is having the right ingredients and seasonings on hand.

In the previous chapters, we talked about some handy kitchen utensils that make producing gluten-free meals a breeze. That's the same with these foods. They allow you to whip up great meals without effort. Some of these foods you'll need to eat and replace weekly; others keep for months. The more you experiment with the recipes, meals, and snacks that work for you, the better sense you'll have of what you need to shop for.

One thing you'll notice is the proliferation of gluten-free foods available at the neighborhood grocery store (not to mention restaurants and bakeries). But if you're looking for more guidance on locating gluten-free-friendly brands, these online resources may come in handy:

- **AMERICANCELIAC.ORG** (American Celiac Disease Alliance)
- **CELIACCENTRAL.ORG** (National Foundation for Celiac Awareness)
- **CELIAC.ORG** (Celiac Disease Foundation)
- **CSACELIACS.ORG** (Celiac Support Association)
- **GLUTENFREELIVING.COM** (*Gluten-Free Living* magazine)
- **GLUTEN.NET** (Gluten Intolerance Group of North America)
- **LIVINGWITHOUT.COM** (*Living Without* magazine)

Gluten-Free Pantry and Shopping List

BAKING ESSENTIALS

- __ Cornstarch
- __ Baking soda
- __ Sugar
- __ Gluten-free pancake/waffle mix
- __ Cornmeal
- __ Vanilla extract
- __ Gluten-free all-purpose flour (a blend of flours)
- __ Baking powder
- __ Xanthan gum or guar gum
- __ Gluten-free baking mixes (such as breads, cakes, cookies, and brownies)

DAIRY

- __ Milk
- __ Buttermilk
- __ Plain cream cheese
- __ Plain yogurt
- __ Greek yogurt
- __ Dairy-free milks
- __ Cheese (not processed)
- __ Eggs and egg substitute

GRAINS, CEREALS, PASTA, AND RICE

__ Amaranth
__ Flaxseed
__ White, wild, and brown rice (plain)
__ Gluten-free corn tortillas
__ Gluten-free waffles

__ Buckwheat
__ Millet
__ Gluten-free cold and hot cereals
__ Gluten-free bread, sandwich buns, rolls

__ Cornmeal or plain grits
__ Quinoa
__ Corn, bean, potato, quinoa, rice, and soy pastas
__ Gluten-free cereal bars

MEAT, FISH, POULTRY, AND MEATLESS PROTEIN SOURCES

__ Fresh or frozen (plain and not injected with broth)
__ Gluten-free deli meats

__ Plain nuts
__ Peanut and other nut butters

__ Dried beans and lentils
__ Canned beans and lentils
__ Tofu (plain)

CONDIMENTS, SAUCES, AND SPICES

__ Ketchup
__ Mayonnaise
__ Mustard (plain)
__ Relish
__ Honey and molasses
__ Hummus

__ Guacamole
__ Jams and jellies
__ Gelatin
__ Vinegar
__ Lower-sodium gluten-free soy sauce

__ Assorted spices (see page 44)
__ Tomato sauce
__ Gluten-free stock and broth
__ Gluten-free sauce packets
__ Gluten-free seasoning packets

FRUITS AND VEGETABLES

__ Fresh or frozen

__ Dried

__ Canned (in juice or water)

FATS AND OILS

__ Butter or buttery spread

__ Vegetable, olive, and canola oils

BREAKFAST

BREAKFAST IS AN IMPORTANT MEAL—AND ONE OF THE TASTIEST. In this chapter, you'll find an assortment of recipes that will hopefully offer you something new to add to your morning rotation, whether you're looking for quick breakfasts for busy weekdays or dishes for more relaxed weekend meals.

Peppery Potato Omelet

1½   **pounds Yukon gold potatoes, peeled and cut into ½-inch pieces**

1   **large red bell pepper**

1   **tablespoon extra-virgin olive oil**

2½   **cups thinly vertically sliced onion**

3   **large eggs, lightly beaten**

3   **large egg whites, lightly beaten**

1   **teaspoon kosher salt, divided**

¼   **teaspoon freshly ground black pepper**

1   **tablespoon chopped fresh parsley**

1. Preheat broiler.

2. Place potatoes in a saucepan; cover with water. Bring to a boil. Reduce heat; simmer 8 minutes or until tender. Drain well.

3. Cut bell pepper in half lengthwise; discard seeds and membranes. Place bell pepper halves, skin sides up, on a foil-lined baking sheet; flatten with hand. Broil 8 minutes or until blackened. Place pepper halves in a paper bag; fold to close tightly. Let stand 10 minutes. Peel and chop.

4. Reduce oven temperature to 350°.

5. Heat a large nonstick ovenproof skillet over medium-high heat. Add oil. Add onion; sauté 5 minutes. Combine eggs, egg whites, and ½ teaspoon salt in a large bowl; stir with a whisk. Pour egg mixture over onions; top with potatoes. Sprinkle potatoes with bell pepper, ½ teaspoon salt, and black pepper. Cook 2 minutes, shaking pan. Place pan in oven; bake at 350° for 8 minutes or until eggs are set. Sprinkle with parsley.

YIELD | SERVES 8 (SERVING SIZE: 1 WEDGE)

CALORIES 149; FAT 3.8g (sat 0.9g, mono 2g, poly 0.6g); PROTEIN 6g; CARB 23g; FIBER 3g; CHOL 70mg; IRON 1mg; SODIUM 295mg; CALC 32mg

Mushroom Frittata

- 2 ounces finely grated fresh pecorino Romano cheese (about ½ cup)
- ¼ teaspoon freshly ground black pepper
- 8 large eggs
- ½ teaspoon salt, divided
- 1 tablespoon extra-virgin olive oil, divided
- 1 (8-ounce) package sliced mushrooms
- ¾ cup chopped green onions
- ⅓ cup chopped fresh basil
- 2 cups baby arugula
- 2 teaspoons lemon juice

1. Preheat oven to 350°.

2. Combine first 3 ingredients; add ¼ teaspoon salt, stirring with a whisk. Heat a 10-inch ovenproof skillet over medium-high heat. Add 2 teaspoons oil; swirl to coat. Add mushrooms and ¼ teaspoon salt; sauté 6 minutes or until mushrooms brown and most of liquid evaporates. Stir in onions; sauté 2 minutes. Reduce heat to medium. Add egg mixture and basil to pan, stirring gently to distribute vegetable mixture; cook 5 minutes or until eggs are partially set. Place pan in oven. Bake at 350° for 7 minutes or until eggs are cooked through and top is lightly browned. Remove pan from oven; let stand 5 minutes. Run a spatula around edge and under frittata to loosen from pan; slide frittata onto a plate or cutting board.

3. Combine 1 teaspoon oil, arugula, and lemon juice. Cut frittata into 6 wedges; top with arugula mixture.

YIELD | SERVES 6 (SERVING SIZE: 1 FRITTATA WEDGE AND ABOUT ⅓ CUP ARUGULA MIXTURE)

CALORIES 145; FAT 8.7g (sat 2.5g, mono 4.2g, poly 1.3g); PROTEIN 10g; CARB 4g; FIBER 0g; CHOL 243mg; IRON 2mg; SODIUM 352mg; CALC 87mg

Zucchini and Red Pepper Frittata

1   large red bell pepper
1   tablespoon olive oil
1   large zucchini, thinly sliced (about 2 cups)
4   ounces white cheddar cheese, shredded (about 1 cup)
¾   cup 2% reduced-fat milk or dairy-free alternative
¼   teaspoon salt
¼   teaspoon freshly ground black pepper
4   large eggs, lightly beaten

1. Preheat broiler.
2. Cut bell pepper in half lengthwise; discard seeds and membranes. Place bell pepper halves, skin sides up, on a foil-lined baking sheet; flatten with hand. Broil 8 minutes or until blackened. Place pepper halves in a paper bag; fold to close tightly. Let stand 10 minutes. Peel and slice.
3. Reduce oven temperature to 350°.
4. Heat a 9-inch nonstick ovenproof skillet over medium-high heat. Add oil to pan; swirl to coat. Add zucchini; cook 6 minutes. Stir in bell pepper; reduce heat to medium. Combine cheese and next 4 ingredients (through eggs) in a large bowl. Add to zucchini mixture; cook 2 minutes or until edges are set. Bake at 350° for 16 minutes or until center is set.
5. Let stand 15 minutes. Cut into 6 wedges.

YIELD | SERVES 6 (SERVING SIZE: 1 WEDGE)

CALORIES 175; FAT 12.4g (sat 5.2g, mono 3g, poly 1g); PROTEIN 11g; CARB 6g; FIBER 1g; CHOL 147mg; IRON 1mg; SODIUM 294mg; CALC 201mg

INGREDIENT TIP
Frittata fillings
These easy egg dishes are open to endless interpretations. Feel free to substitute your favorite vegetables and cheeses.

Mexican Chorizo Hash

This breakfast-for-dinner skillet gets heat from spicy Mexican chorizo. Don't stir the potatoes too much as they cook, so they crisp in the pan.

2	ounces Mexican chorizo
1	cup chopped onion
¼	cup coarsely chopped bottled roasted red bell peppers
½	teaspoon kosher salt
½	teaspoon freshly ground black pepper
1	(6-ounce) package baby spinach
2	teaspoons olive oil
2½	cups refrigerated gluten-free shredded hash brown potatoes
4	large eggs

1. Heat a large skillet over medium-high heat. Add chorizo to pan; cook 3 minutes or until browned, stirring to crumble. Add onion, bell pepper, salt, and black pepper; cook 3 minutes, stirring occasionally. Add spinach; stir until spinach wilts. Remove sausage mixture from pan. Add oil to pan; swirl to coat. Add potatoes; cook 8 minutes or until bottom is crisp. Stir in sausage mixture. Make 4 egg-sized spaces in pan with a spoon. Crack 1 egg into each space. Cover and cook 4 minutes or until egg yolks are slightly set.

YIELD | SERVES 4 (SERVING SIZE: ABOUT 1 CUP POTATO MIXTURE AND 1 EGG)

CALORIES 279; **FAT** 11.1g (sat 3.9g, mono 3.5g, poly 1.2g); **PROTEIN** 13g; **CARB** 33g; **FIBER** 5g; **CHOL** 206mg; **IRON** 2mg; **SODIUM** 616mg; **CALC** 68mg

Cheesy Hash Brown Casserole

1 cup gluten-free unsalted chicken stock
2 cups chopped onion, divided
2 (8-ounce) packages presliced white mushrooms, divided
6 garlic cloves
½ cup light sour cream
4 ounces reduced-fat sharp cheddar cheese, shredded and divided (about 1 cup)
1 teaspoon freshly ground black pepper
½ teaspoon kosher salt
3 center-cut bacon slices
1 (30-ounce) package frozen gluten-free shredded hash brown potatoes, thawed
1 tablespoon olive oil, divided
2 large eggs, lightly beaten
2 ounces 40%-less-fat original kettle-style potato chips, crushed
3 tablespoons chopped fresh flat-leaf parsley

1. Preheat oven to 400°.

2. Combine stock, 1 cup onion, half of mushrooms, and garlic in a saucepan; bring to a boil. Cover, reduce heat, and simmer 10 minutes or until mushrooms are tender. Place mixture in a blender. Remove center piece of lid (to allow steam to escape); secure blender lid on blender. Place a towel over opening in lid (to avoid splatters); blend until smooth. Stir in sour cream, 2 ounces cheese, pepper, and salt; blend until smooth.

3. Cook bacon in a large cast-iron skillet over medium heat until crisp. Remove bacon from pan; crumble. Add half of potatoes to drippings in pan; cover and cook 4 minutes on each side or until browned. Remove potatoes from pan. Repeat procedure with remaining potatoes and 2 teaspoons oil. Remove from pan.

4. Add 1 teaspoon oil to pan; swirl to coat. Add 1 cup onion and remaining mushrooms; cook 6 minutes or until tender. Return potatoes to pan; add eggs, stirring well to combine. Pour sour cream mixture over potato mixture. Sprinkle with bacon, 2 ounces cheese, chips, and parsley. Bake at 400° for 10 minutes or until cheese melts. Turn broiler on (do not remove pan from oven); broil 1½ minutes or until lightly browned.

YIELD | SERVES 8 (SERVING SIZE: 1 WEDGE)

CALORIES 273; FAT 9.7g (sat 4g, mono 2.9g, poly 0.7g); PROTEIN 13g; CARB 34g; FIBER 3g; CHOL 63mg; IRON 1mg; SODIUM 379mg; CALC 178mg

Sunflower Granola

1	cup certified gluten-free old-fashioned rolled oats
¼	cup raw sunflower seed kernels
¼	cup shredded sweetened coconut
¼	cup chopped walnuts
¼	cup flaxseed meal
½	teaspoon ground cinnamon
¼	teaspoon salt
2	tablespoons butter, melted
2	tablespoons honey
½	teaspoon vanilla extract

1. Place oven rack on middle shelf, about 10 inches below broiler. Preheat broiler.

2. Combine first 7 ingredients on a baking sheet; toss well. Broil 3 minutes or until lightly toasted, stirring every 1 minute. Combine butter, honey, and vanilla in a small bowl. Drizzle butter mixture over oat mixture; toss to coat. Broil 2 minutes or until well toasted, stirring after 1 minute. Remove granola from oven; cool on pan 8 minutes, stirring occasionally.

YIELD | SERVES 8 (SERVING SIZE: ¼ CUP)

CALORIES 159; FAT 10.4g (sat 3.3g, mono 2.4g, poly 4g); PROTEIN 4g; CARB 15g; FIBER 3g; CHOL 8mg; IRON 1mg; SODIUM 107mg; CALC 15mg

Pumpkinseed-Almond Granola

½	cup certified gluten-free old-fashioned rolled oats
¼	cup unsalted pumpkinseed kernels, roasted
1	ounce lightly salted smoked almonds, chopped
5	teaspoons brown sugar
1½	tablespoons canola oil
1	teaspoon grated orange rind
1	tablespoon fresh orange juice
¼	teaspoon vanilla extract
⅛	teaspoon salt

1. Preheat oven to 325°.

2. Combine all ingredients in a medium bowl, stirring well with a spatula. Spread mixture on a parchment paper–lined baking sheet. Bake at 325° for 26 minutes. Cool completely.

YIELD | SERVES 4

CALORIES 195; FAT 13.4g (sat 1.4g, mono 6.9g, poly 4g); PROTEIN 5g; CARB 16g; FIBER 2g; CHOL 0mg; IRON 1mg; SODIUM 107mg; CALC 24mg

Vanilla Amaranth with Peach Compote

2   teaspoons butter
1   cup uncooked amaranth
2   cups 1% low-fat milk or dairy-free alternative
Dash of salt
½   vanilla bean (split lengthwise)
¾   pound sliced peaches (fresh or frozen)
¼   cup water
2   tablespoons sugar
⅛   teaspoon ground cinnamon
Dash of ground ginger

1. Melt butter in a medium saucepan over medium heat. Add amaranth; cook 2 minutes. Stir in milk, dash of salt, and vanilla bean; bring to a boil. Cover, reduce heat, and simmer 20 minutes or until liquid is absorbed. Discard vanilla bean.

2. Combine peaches, ¼ cup water, sugar, cinnamon, and dash of ground ginger in a saucepan over medium-high heat; bring to a boil. Simmer 12 minutes or until peaches are tender and thick. Serve peaches over amaranth.

YIELD | SERVES 4 (SERVING SIZE: ½ CUP AMARANTH AND ⅓ CUP FRUIT)

CALORIES 310; FAT 6.7g (sat 2.7g, mono 1.7g, poly 1.5g); PROTEIN 11g; CARB 53g; FIBER 5g; CHOL 0mg; IRON 0mg; SODIUM 58mg; CALC 0mg

Savory Buckwheat with Tomato, Cheddar, and Bacon

This gluten-free, polenta-like cereal packs 41 grams of whole grains into one serving.

⅔   cup cooked cereal (such as Bob's Red Mill Creamy Buckwheat Hot Cereal)
1   center-cut bacon slice, cooked and crumbled
2   tablespoons reduced-fat shredded cheddar cheese
2   tablespoons chopped tomato
     Slivered jalapeño pepper

1. Top cooked cereal with cooked and crumbled bacon, shredded cheddar cheese, chopped tomato, and slivered jalapeño pepper.

YIELD | SERVES 1

CALORIES 194; FAT 4g (sat 1.6g, mono 0.3g, poly 0.1g); PROTEIN 11g; CARB 31g; FIBER 3g; CHOL 10mg; IRON 1mg; SODIUM 223mg; CALC 101mg

Quinoa with Strawberries and Buttermilk

¾   cup cooked quinoa (such as Ancient Harvest Traditional Organic)
¼   cup low-fat buttermilk
½   cup sliced strawberries
2   tablespoons sliced almonds, toasted
1   teaspoon honey

1. Combine cooked quinoa and buttermilk in a microwave-safe bowl. Microwave at HIGH 45 seconds. Stir; let stand 1 minute. Top with sliced strawberries, almonds, and honey.

YIELD | SERVES 1

CALORIES 305; FAT 9.1g (sat 0.8g, mono 3.7g, poly 1.5g); PROTEIN 11g; CARB 47g; FIBER 7g; CHOL 2mg; IRON 3mg; SODIUM 75mg; CALC 139mg

Breakfast Quinoa

Like most whole grains, quinoa is surprisingly filling, but if you need more for breakfast, serve with an egg on the side.

½   cup uncooked quinoa
¾   cup light coconut milk
2   tablespoons water
1   tablespoon brown sugar
⅛   teaspoon salt
¼   cup flaked unsweetened coconut
1   cup sliced strawberries
1   cup sliced banana

1. Preheat oven to 400°.
2. Place quinoa in a fine sieve, and place the sieve in a large bowl. Cover quinoa with water. Using your hands, rub grains together 30 seconds; rinse and drain quinoa. Repeat procedure twice. Drain well. Combine quinoa, coconut milk, 2 tablespoons water, brown sugar, and salt in a medium saucepan; bring to a boil. Reduce heat, and simmer 15 minutes or until liquid is absorbed, stirring occasionally. Stir mixture constantly during the last 2 minutes of cooking.
3. While quinoa cooks, spread flaked coconut in a single layer on a baking sheet. Bake at 400° for 5 minutes or until golden brown. Cool slightly.
4. Place about ½ cup quinoa mixture in each of 4 bowls. Top each serving with ¼ cup strawberry slices, ¼ cup banana slices, and 1 tablespoon toasted coconut. Serve warm.

YIELD | SERVES 4

CALORIES 178; FAT 5.5g (sat 3.8g, mono 0.4g, poly 0.8g); PROTEIN 4g; CARB 30g; FIBER 4g; CHOL 0mg; IRON 2mg; SODIUM 89mg; CALC 22mg

Oatmeal Pancakes

Now that potato starch and flours like tapioca flour are more widely available, it's easy to make your own gluten-free mix from scratch and have this mix on hand for whenever the urge for pancakes or waffles strikes.

Oatmeal Pancake and Waffle Mix:
- 4 ounces certified gluten-free oat flour (about 1 cup)
- 2.7 ounces potato starch (about ½ cup)
- 1.1 ounces tapioca flour (about ¼ cup)
- 2 tablespoons sugar
- 2 tablespoons baking powder
- 1 tablespoon flaxseed meal
- 2 teaspoons baking soda
- ⅛ teaspoon salt
- ½ cup certified gluten-free old-fashioned rolled oats

Remaining ingredients:
- 1½ cups low-fat buttermilk
- ¼ cup butter, melted
- 2 large egg whites, beaten

1. To prepare Oatmeal Pancake and Waffle Mix, weigh or lightly spoon oat flour, potato starch, and tapioca flour into dry measuring cups; level with a knife. Combine flours, potato starch, and next 5 ingredients (through salt) in a medium bowl, stirring well with a whisk. Add oats, stirring with a whisk.

2. Combine buttermilk, butter, and egg whites; add to mix, stirring until smooth. Pour ¼ cup batter per pancake onto a hot nonstick griddle or nonstick skillet. Cook 1 to 2 minutes or until tops are covered with bubbles and edges look cooked. Carefully turn pancakes over; cook 1 to 2 minutes or until bottoms are lightly browned.

YIELD | SERVES 7 (SERVING SIZE: 2 PANCAKES)

CALORIES 242; FAT 9.2g (sat 4.6g, mono 2.8g, poly 1.8g); PROTEIN 7g; CARB 33g; FIBER 3g; CHOL 20mg; IRON 1mg; SODIUM 355mg; CALC 143mg

Blueberry-Almond Oatmeal Pancakes

These blueberry pancakes get a double dose of almond flavor from the nuts and almond extract. Almond extract can be bitter when used in excess, so don't be tempted to add more—this amount is just right. If fresh blueberries are in season, feel free to substitute them for the frozen called for in the recipe.

2½ cups Oatmeal Pancake and Waffle Mix (page 80)
1½ cups low-fat buttermilk
¼   cup butter, melted
2   tablespoons maple syrup
¼   teaspoon almond extract
2   large egg whites, beaten
1   cup frozen small blueberries
1   tablespoon certified gluten-free oat flour
½   cup sliced almonds, toasted
1¼ cups maple syrup

1. Lightly spoon mix into dry measuring cups; level with a knife. Place mix in a large bowl. Combine buttermilk and next 4 ingredients (through egg whites), stirring with a whisk; add to mix, stirring until smooth. Let stand 10 minutes.

2. Combine blueberries and oat flour, tossing to coat. Fold blueberry mixture and almonds into batter.

3. Pour about ¼ cup batter per pancake onto a hot nonstick griddle or nonstick skillet. Cook 2 to 3 minutes or until tops are covered with bubbles and edges look cooked. Carefully turn pancakes over; cook 2 to 3 minutes or until bottoms are lightly browned. Serve with maple syrup.

YIELD | SERVES 10 (SERVING SIZE: 2 PANCAKES AND 2 TABLESPOONS SYRUP)

CALORIES 319; FAT 8.9g (sat 3.4g, mono 3.2g, poly 1.8g); PROTEIN 6g; CARB 56g; FIBER 3g; CHOL 14mg; IRON 1mg; SODIUM 254mg; CALC 157mg

Pecan-Oatmeal Waffles

Toasted pecans add a nutty sweetness to these oatmeal waffles flavored with cinnamon. Topped with sliced bananas and strawberries, with a swirl of maple syrup for added sweetness, they make a festive, pretty breakfast for your family or brunch for a crowd.

2½ cups Oatmeal Pancake and Waffle Mix (page 80)
¼   teaspoon ground cinnamon
1½ cups low-fat buttermilk
¼   cup butter, melted
2   tablespoons maple syrup
1   teaspoon vanilla extract
2   large egg whites, beaten
⅓   cup chopped pecans, toasted
Cooking spray
1   cup (⅛-inch-thick) slices banana
1   cup sliced strawberries
½   cup maple syrup

1. Lightly spoon mix into dry measuring cups; level with a knife. Combine mix and cinnamon in a large bowl, stirring with a whisk. Combine buttermilk and next 4 ingredients (through egg whites), stirring with a whisk; add to mix, stirring until smooth. Fold in pecans. Let stand 10 minutes.

2. Coat a round waffle iron with cooking spray; preheat.

3. Spoon about ½ cup batter per waffle onto hot waffle iron, spreading batter to edges. Cook 1½ minutes or until steaming stops; repeat procedure with remaining batter. Top waffles with banana and strawberry slices. Serve with syrup.

YIELD | SERVES 8 (SERVING SIZE: 1 WAFFLE, ABOUT ¼ CUP FRUIT, AND 1 TABLESPOON SYRUP)

CALORIES 336; FAT 11.7g (sat 4.4g, mono 4.2g, poly 2.1g); PROTEIN 6g; CARB 53g; FIBER 4g; CHOL 17mg; IRON 1mg; SODIUM 315mg; CALC 159mg

Mixed Berry Muffins

3.45 ounces brown rice flour (about ¾ cup)
2.6 ounces potato starch (about ½ cup)
1.8 ounces certified gluten-free oat flour (about ½ cup)
⅓   cup granulated sugar
¼   cup packed brown sugar
1½   teaspoons baking powder
1   teaspoon xanthan gum
½   teaspoon salt
½   cup 1% low-fat milk or dairy-free alternative
¼   cup butter, melted
2   large eggs
1½   cups mixed fresh berries (such as blueberries, raspberries, and blackberries)
Cooking spray
1   tablespoon turbinado sugar or granulated sugar

1. Preheat oven to 350°.

2. Weigh or lightly spoon brown rice flour, potato starch, and oat flour into dry measuring cups; level with a knife. Combine brown rice flour, potato starch, oat flour, granulated sugar, and next 4 ingredients (through salt) in a medium bowl; stir with a whisk. Make a well in center of mixture. Combine milk, butter, and eggs, and stir with a whisk. Add to flour mixture, stirring just until moist. Fold in berries.

3. Place 12 paper muffin cup liners in muffin cups; coat liners with cooking spray. Spoon batter into prepared cups, and sprinkle with turbinado sugar. Bake at 350° for 25 minutes or until lightly browned and muffins spring back when lightly touched. Cool 10 minutes in pan on a wire rack; remove from pan.

Note: If you're planning to freeze all or some of the muffins, leave off the turbinado sugar.

YIELD | SERVES 12 (SERVING SIZE: 1 MUFFIN)

CALORIES 172; FAT 5.6g (sat 3g, mono 1.7g, poly 0.6g); PROTEIN 3g; CARB 28g; FIBER 2g; CHOL 42mg; IRON 1mg; SODIUM 206mg; CALC 70mg

INGREDIENT TIP

Oat flour If you can't find oat flour in your grocery store, make your own. Just place certified gluten-free oats in a food processor, and grind into a powdery consistency.

Cinnamon, Apple, and Oat Scones

4.2 ounces sweet white sorghum flour (about 1 cup)

1.3 ounces white rice flour (about ¼ cup)

1.2 ounces brown rice flour (about ¼ cup)

1.3 ounces potato starch (about ¼ cup)

1 cup certified gluten-free quick-cooking oats

¼ cup packed brown sugar

2 teaspoons baking powder

1 teaspoon xanthan gum

1 teaspoon baking soda

½ teaspoon salt

½ teaspoon ground cinnamon

¼ teaspoon ground nutmeg

5 tablespoons chilled unsalted butter, cut into small pieces

1 cup finely diced, peeled Granny Smith apple

¼ cup cinnamon-flavored baking chips

½ cup low-fat buttermilk

¼ cup applesauce

White rice flour, for dusting

1 egg white, lightly beaten

2 teaspoons turbinado sugar or granulated sugar

1. Preheat oven to 400°.

2. Weigh or lightly spoon flours and potato starch into dry measuring cups; level with a knife. Combine flours, potato starch, oats, and next 7 ingredients (through nutmeg), stirring with a whisk; cut in butter with a pastry blender or 2 knives until mixture resembles coarse meal. Stir in apple and baking chips. Add buttermilk and applesauce; stir just until moist.

3. Turn dough out onto a surface lightly dusted with white rice flour. Pat dough into an 8-inch circle; cut into 14 wedges. Place wedges on a baking sheet lined with parchment paper. Brush egg white over surface of dough; sprinkle with turbinado sugar. Bake at 400° for 14 minutes or until golden brown. Serve warm.

Note: If you're planning to freeze all or some of the scones, leave off the turbinado sugar.

YIELD | SERVES 14 (SERVING SIZE: 1 SCONE)

CALORIES 169; FAT 6.1g (sat 3.3g, mono 1.3g, poly 0.3g); PROTEIN 3g; CARB 26g; FIBER 2g; CHOL 11mg; IRON 1mg; SODIUM 269mg; CALC 67mg

LUNCH IS OFTEN A MEAL GRABBED ON THE GO OR EATEN AT YOUR DESK.

It might also consist of leftovers that you're not exactly looking forward to. The goal with this chapter is to offer you some fresh ideas to make your midday meal something a little more special.

Salmon Salad on Arugula

One serving of this tasty fresh fish salad packs in a full day's worth of omega-3 fatty acids. Keep refrigerated in an airtight container up to two days.

- 4   **(6-ounce) salmon fillets, skinned**
- ¼   **teaspoon kosher salt**
- ¼   **teaspoon black pepper**
- 2   **tablespoons olive oil, divided**
- 2   **tablespoons fresh lemon juice, divided**
- 2   **tablespoons plain fat-free Greek yogurt**
- 2   **tablespoons crème fraîche or sour cream**
- 2   **tablespoons thinly sliced fresh basil**
- 4   **teaspoons capers, rinsed, drained, and chopped**
- 4   **cups baby arugula leaves**
- 1   **cup very thinly vertically sliced red onion**

1. Sprinkle salmon with salt and pepper. Heat a medium nonstick skillet over medium-high heat. Add 1 tablespoon oil to pan; swirl to coat. Add salmon; cook 6 minutes on each side or until fish flakes easily when tested with a fork or until desired degree of doneness. Cool to room temperature; flake with a fork.

2. Combine salmon, 1 tablespoon juice, yogurt, and next 3 ingredients (through capers) in a medium bowl. Refrigerate 30 minutes or up to 3 hours.

3. Combine 1 tablespoon oil, 1 tablespoon juice, arugula, and onion in a bowl. Toss gently to coat. Divide arugula mixture among 4 plates. Top with salmon mixture.

YIELD | SERVES 4 (SERVING SIZE: 1 CUP ARUGULA AND ⅔ CUP SALMON MIXTURE)

CALORIES 354; FAT 19.4g (sat 4.6g, mono 8.6g, poly 4g); PROTEIN 38g; CARB 5g; FIBER 1g; CHOL 97mg; IRON 1mg; SODIUM 297mg; CALC 65mg

Spicy Bean and Quinoa Salad with "Mole" Vinaigrette

To make this salad ahead, leave out the greens and keep the quinoa mixture covered in the refrigerator up to two days. Add the spinach just before serving.

- 1 teaspoon grated orange rind
- 2 tablespoons fresh orange juice
- 1½ tablespoons red wine vinegar
- 1 tablespoon adobo sauce from canned chipotle chiles in adobo sauce
- ¾ teaspoon unsweetened cocoa
- ½ teaspoon ground cumin
- ½ teaspoon ground cinnamon
- 2 tablespoons olive oil
- 3 cups cooked quinoa, at room temperature
- ½ cup unsalted pumpkinseed kernels, toasted
- ¼ cup chopped fresh cilantro
- ½ teaspoon kosher salt
- 2 green onions, thinly sliced
- 1 Fresno chile or jalapeño pepper, very thinly sliced
- 1 (15-ounce) can black beans, rinsed and drained
- 4 cups baby spinach leaves

1. Combine first 7 ingredients in a bowl; gradually add oil, stirring well with a whisk.

2. Combine quinoa and next 6 ingredients (through beans) in a large bowl. Add vinaigrette; toss to coat. Add spinach; toss to combine.

YIELD | SERVES 6 (SERVING SIZE: 1⅔ CUPS)

CALORIES 258; FAT 11.6g (sat 1.5g, mono 5.2g, poly 2.4g); PROTEIN 10g; CARB 31g; FIBER 7g; CHOL 0mg; IRON 4mg; SODIUM 377mg; CALC 55mg

Warm Brown Rice and Chickpea Salad with Cherries and Goat Cheese

Fresh cherries add a meaty bite and tart-sweet flavor. If you can't find fresh cherries, add 2 tablespoons boiling water to ¼ cup unsweetened dried cherries. Let stand 10 minutes; drain and chop.

1 (8.8-ounce) pouch precooked brown rice (such as Uncle Ben's)
¼ cup chopped green onions
¼ cup chopped fresh basil
3 tablespoons extra-virgin olive oil
2 tablespoons white balsamic vinegar
½ teaspoon salt
¼ teaspoon freshly ground black pepper
32 cherries, pitted and quartered
1 (15-ounce) can unsalted chickpeas, rinsed and drained
2 ounces crumbled goat cheese (about ½ cup)

1. Heat rice according to package directions. Place rice in a medium bowl. Stir in onions and next 7 ingredients (through chickpeas). Sprinkle with goat cheese.

YIELD | SERVES 4 (SERVING SIZE: 1 CUP)

CALORIES 359; FAT 16.8g (sat 4.6g, mono 8.4g, poly 1.2g); PROTEIN 10g; CARB 43g; FIBER 5g; CHOL 11mg; IRON 2mg; SODIUM 389mg; CALC 100mg

Roasted Carrot, Chicken, and Grape Quinoa Bowl

- 2 cups (¾-inch) diagonally cut carrot
- 2 teaspoons olive oil
- ½ teaspoon kosher salt, divided
- Cooking spray
- 5 tablespoons plain 2% reduced-fat Greek yogurt
- 3 tablespoons fresh lemon juice
- 2 tablespoons water
- 1½ tablespoons honey
- ¾ teaspoon ground cumin
- ½ teaspoon freshly ground black pepper
- 1½ cups cooked quinoa
- 1½ cups shredded skinless, boneless rotisserie chicken breast
- 1½ cups seedless red grapes, halved
- ½ cup thinly sliced green onions
- ½ cup fresh flat-leaf parsley leaves
- ½ cup sliced almonds, toasted
- 4 cups mixed salad greens

1. Preheat oven to 450°.

2. Combine carrot, oil, and ¼ teaspoon salt on a jelly-roll pan coated with cooking spray; toss to coat. Bake at 450° for 15 minutes or until tender.

3. Combine ¼ teaspoon salt, yogurt, and next 5 ingredients (through pepper) in a large bowl, stirring with a whisk. Add carrot, quinoa, and next 5 ingredients (through almonds); toss. Place 1 cup salad greens in each of 4 shallow bowls; top each serving with about 1½ cups quinoa mixture.

YIELD | SERVES 4

CALORIES 371; FAT 12.3g (sat 1.6g, mono 6.2g, poly 2g); PROTEIN 25g; CARB 44g; FIBER 7g; CHOL 51mg; IRON 3mg; SODIUM 502mg; CALC 142mg

Blueberry Chicken Salad

12 ounces shredded skinless, boneless rotisserie chicken (about 3 cups)
½ cup thinly vertically sliced red onion
⅓ cup diced celery
¼ cup torn fresh basil
½ teaspoon kosher salt, divided
½ cup plain 2% reduced-fat Greek yogurt
2½ tablespoons fresh lemon juice, divided
1 tablespoon honey
2 cups fresh blueberries
1 (5-ounce) package baby arugula
2 teaspoons extra-virgin olive oil
¼ teaspoon freshly ground black pepper

1. Combine first 4 ingredients in a medium bowl; sprinkle with ¼ teaspoon salt. Combine yogurt, 1 tablespoon lemon juice, and honey in a small bowl, stirring with a whisk. Add yogurt mixture to chicken mixture; toss to coat. Gently stir in blueberries. Place arugula, 1½ tablespoons lemon juice, oil, ¼ teaspoon salt, and pepper in a bowl; toss to coat. Divide arugula mixture among 6 plates; top each serving with about ¾ cup chicken mixture.

YIELD | SERVES 6

CALORIES 188; FAT 8.5g (sat 2.1g, mono 3.9g, poly 1.3g); PROTEIN 16g; CARB 13g; FIBER 2g; CHOL 75mg; IRON 1mg; SODIUM 369mg; CALC 69mg

Tuna-Pecan Salad Sandwiches

⅓ cup chopped celery
⅓ cup diced Gala apple (about 1 small)
⅓ cup fat-free mayonnaise
¼ cup chopped pecans, toasted
¼ teaspoon salt
¼ teaspoon freshly ground black pepper
1 (12-ounce) can albacore tuna in water, drained
4 curly leaf lettuce leaves
4 gluten-free English muffins, split and toasted

1. Combine first 7 ingredients in a small bowl. Place a lettuce leaf on half of each English muffin. Top with tuna salad. Top with remaining English muffin halves.

YIELD | SERVES 4 (SERVING SIZE: 1 SANDWICH)

CALORIES 302; FAT 9.5 (sat 1g, mono 3.7g, poly 3.6g); PROTEIN 18g; CARB 47g; FIBER 4g; CHOL 18mg; IRON 4mg; SODIUM 752mg; CALC 19mg

Spicy Steak Lettuce Wraps

These wraps give traditional lettuce wraps a kick in the taste buds with the addition of zesty-spiced steak.

- 1 (12-ounce) sirloin steak, trimmed
- 2 tablespoons dark brown sugar
- 3 tablespoons rice vinegar
- 3 tablespoons gluten-free lower-sodium soy sauce
- 2 tablespoons grated shallots
- 2 tablespoons sambal oelek (ground fresh chile paste)
- 1 tablespoon grated peeled fresh ginger
- 2 teaspoons sesame oil
- Cooking spray
- 12 large Boston lettuce leaves (about 2 heads)
- 1 cup matchstick-cut English cucumber
- 1 cup thinly sliced red onion
- 1 cup matchstick-cut carrots
- ½ cup fresh cilantro leaves

1. Place steak in freezer 15 minutes. Remove from freezer; cut across grain into ⅛-inch-thick slices. Combine sugar and next 6 ingredients (through oil) in a large zip-top plastic bag; seal bag, and shake. Remove 3 tablespoons marinade, and set aside. Add steak to marinade in bag; seal and shake. Marinate in refrigerator 1 hour. Remove steak from bag; discard marinade. Heat a large skillet over medium-high heat. Coat pan with cooking spray. Add steak to pan, and cook 1 minute on each side.

2. Divide steak among lettuce leaves. Top each leaf with 4 teaspoons cucumber, 4 teaspoons onion, 4 teaspoons carrots, and 2 teaspoons cilantro; drizzle with reserved 3 tablespoons marinade.

YIELD | SERVES 4 (SERVING SIZE: 3 LETTUCE WRAPS)

CALORIES 268; FAT 13.5g (sat 4.7g, mono 5.6g, poly 1.5g); PROTEIN 19g; CARB 18g; FIBER 2g; CHOL 64mg; IRON 2mg; SODIUM 363mg; CALC 57mg

Pork Wraps with Fresh Tomatillo Salsa

2 large tomatillos
½ cup chopped cucumber
¼ cup chopped fresh cilantro
2 tablespoons fresh lime juice
½ teaspoon salt, divided
1 garlic clove, peeled
Cooking spray
1 pound boneless pork cutlets, cut into thin strips
1 teaspoon ground cumin
2 medium poblano chiles, stemmed, seeded, and cut into thin strips
1 medium onion, vertically sliced
4 (8-inch) gluten-free tortillas
½ cup light sour cream

INGREDIENT TIP

Warming tortillas

Since gluten-free tortillas are stored in the refrigerator, they'll need to be warmed to prevent breaking. You can steam them by placing each tortilla on a splatter guard set over a pan of simmering water. Cover with a lid, and heat about 5 to 10 seconds or until they're soft and pliable. Or you can warm them in the microwave (see page 103 for instructions).

1. Discard husks and stems from tomatillos. Place tomatillos, cucumber, cilantro, lime juice, ¼ teaspoon salt, and garlic in a blender. Process until finely chopped, and set aside.

2. Heat a large nonstick skillet over medium-high heat. Coat pan with cooking spray. Sprinkle pork with cumin. Add pork to pan; cook 3 minutes or until no longer pink in center, stirring occasionally. Remove from pan; keep warm.

3. Recoat pan with cooking spray; add chiles and onion. Coat vegetables with cooking spray; cook 4 minutes or until onion begins to brown, stirring frequently.

4. While vegetables cook, warm tortillas.

5. Return pork to pan; add ¼ teaspoon salt, and cook 30 seconds or until pork mixture is thoroughly heated, stirring constantly.

6. Divide pork mixture among tortillas. Top each with about ⅓ cup salsa; roll up. Serve with sour cream.

YIELD | SERVES 4 (SERVING SIZE: 1 WRAP AND 2 TABLESPOONS SOUR CREAM)

CALORIES 350; FAT 10.1g (sat 3.2g, mono 2.9g, poly 2.4g); PROTEIN 29g; CARB 36g; FIBER 6g; CHOL 85mg; IRON 3mg; SODIUM 468mg; CALC 57mg

Spicy Chicken Sandwiches

¼ cup reduced-fat mayonnaise

2 tablespoons chopped fresh cilantro

1 teaspoon fresh lime juice

1 garlic clove, minced

2 egg whites, lightly beaten

3 tablespoons hot pepper sauce (such as Tabasco)

1 teaspoon dried oregano

½ teaspoon salt

2 (6-ounce) skinless, boneless chicken breast halves

4½ ounces gluten-free tortilla chips (about 6 cups)

2 tablespoons olive oil

4 (1.5-ounce) gluten-free sandwich rolls

12 (⅛-inch-thick) slices red onion

4 lettuce leaves

1. Combine first 4 ingredients; refrigerate until ready to prepare sandwiches.

2. Combine egg whites and next 3 ingredients (through salt) in a large zip-top plastic bag. Cut chicken breast halves in half horizontally to form 4 cutlets. Add chicken to bag; seal. Marinate in refrigerator at least 2 hours or up to 8 hours, turning bag occasionally.

3. Place tortilla chips in a food processor; process 1 minute or until ground. Place ground chips in a shallow dish.

4. Working with 1 cutlet at a time, remove chicken from bag, allowing excess marinade to drip off. Coat chicken completely in chips. Set aside. Repeat procedure with remaining chicken and chips.

5. Heat a large nonstick skillet over medium heat. Add oil to pan, swirling to coat. Add chicken to pan; cook 3 minutes on each side or until browned and done. Spread mayonnaise mixture evenly over cut sides of rolls. Layer bottom half of each roll with 3 onion slices, 1 lettuce leaf, and 1 chicken cutlet; top with top halves of rolls.

YIELD | SERVES 4 (SERVING SIZE: 1 SANDWICH)

CALORIES 416; FAT 10.8g (sat 2g, mono 3.9g, poly 3.4g); PROTEIN 29g; CARB 56g; FIBER 8g; CHOL 54mg; IRON 1mg; SODIUM 802mg; CALC 408mg

Spicy-Sweet Chicken Lettuce Cups

A quick vinegar soak keeps the chicken moist and intensely flavorful in this dish.

2	cups cider vinegar
1	cup water
½	cup sugar
2	tablespoons sliced serrano chile
¾	teaspoon kosher salt
1	small garlic clove, crushed
1	cup matchstick-cut carrots
1½	cups shredded skinless, boneless rotisserie chicken breast
1½	cups shredded skinless, boneless rotisserie chicken thigh or drumstick
12	butter lettuce leaves
24	English cucumber slices
6	tablespoons dry-roasted peanuts, chopped
¼	cup torn fresh mint

1. Combine first 6 ingredients in a medium saucepan. Bring mixture to a boil; cook 20 minutes. Remove from heat. Stir in carrots; let stand 10 minutes to soften. Add chicken to carrot mixture; let stand 5 minutes. Drain and discard liquid.

2. Place about ¼ cup chicken mixture in each lettuce leaf, and top each lettuce leaf with 2 cucumber slices, 1½ teaspoons peanuts, and 1 teaspoon mint.

YIELD | SERVES 6 (SERVING SIZE: 2 LETTUCE CUPS)

CALORIES 147; FAT 7g (sat 1.4g, mono 3.2g, poly 1.6g); PROTEIN 18g; CARB 5g; FIBER 1g; CHOL 58mg; IRON 1mg; SODIUM 265mg; CALC 25mg

INGREDIENT TIP

Dark and light meat

A mix of chicken breast and thigh or drumstick gives these lettuce cups more richness, but feel free to use all white meat, if you prefer.

Chicken-Olive Quesadillas

3	ounces part-skim mozzarella cheese, shredded (about ¾ cup)
½	cup chopped cooked chicken breast
3	tablespoons sliced ripe olives
¼	teaspoon chili powder
¼	teaspoon ground cumin
1	(4-ounce) can chopped green chiles, drained
	Butter-flavored cooking spray
4	(6-inch) corn tortillas
	Fresh salsa (optional)
	Reduced-fat sour cream (optional)

1. Combine first 6 ingredients in a medium bowl.

2. Heat a large nonstick skillet over medium-high heat. Coat pan with cooking spray. Add 1 tortilla to pan. Spread about ½ cup chicken mixture on left half of tortilla; fold right side of tortilla over filling, pressing gently with a spatula. Place an additional tortilla in pan, overlapping first quesadilla. Spread about ½ cup chicken mixture on right half of tortilla; fold left side of tortilla over filling, pressing with spatula. (Folded sides of tortillas should meet in center of pan.) Cook 1 minute.

3. Coat quesadillas with cooking spray; turn quesadillas over, keeping folded sides together in center of pan. Cook 1 to 2 minutes or until golden and cheese melts. Remove from pan; cover and keep warm. Repeat procedure with cooking spray and remaining tortillas and filling. Serve immediately with salsa and sour cream, if desired.

YIELD | SERVES 4 (SERVING SIZE: 1 QUESADILLA)

CALORIES 178; **FAT** 6.3g (sat 1.4g, mono 2.6g, poly 1.8g); **PROTEIN** 12g; **CARB** 16g; **FIBER** 1g; **CHOL** 15mg; **IRON** 0mg; **SODIUM** 312mg; **CALC** 9mg

Portobello and Black Bean Quesadillas

4 (8-inch) gluten-free tortillas
Butter-flavored cooking spray
2 (4½-inch) portobello mushroom caps, chopped
1 cup canned unsalted black beans, rinsed and drained
2 tablespoons light balsamic vinaigrette
1 (2-ounce) jar diced pimiento, drained
4 ounces preshredded reduced-fat 4-cheese Mexican blend cheese
   (about 1 cup)
¼ cup thinly sliced green onions
Fresh salsa (optional)
Reduced-fat sour cream (optional)

1. Stack tortillas; microwave at HIGH 1 minute. Leave in microwave to keep warm while preparing filling.

2. Heat a large nonstick skillet over medium-high heat. Coat pan with cooking spray. Add mushrooms; sauté 2 minutes or until tender. Add beans, vinaigrette, and pimiento; cook 1 to 2 minutes or until liquid evaporates, stirring constantly. Mash bean mixture slightly with a potato masher.

3. Spoon about ⅓ cup bean mixture onto each tortilla. Sprinkle with cheese and onions. Fold tortillas in half.

4. Wipe pan with paper towels; heat over medium heat. Coat pan with cooking spray. Place 2 quesadillas in pan; cook 2 to 3 minutes on each side or until golden and cheese melts. Repeat procedure with remaining 2 quesadillas. Cut each quesadilla into 3 wedges. Serve immediately with salsa and sour cream, if desired.

YIELD | SERVES 4 (SERVING SIZE: 1 QUESADILLA)

CALORIES 289; FAT 9.3g (sat 3.4g, mono 2.2g, poly 1.5g); PROTEIN 14g; CARB 38g; FIBER 6g; CHOL 18mg; IRON 2mg; SODIUM 512mg; CALC 364mg

Broccoli-Cheese Soup

Traditional broccoli-cheese soup has nearly 400 calories and more than 18 grams of saturated fat per serving. Ours has fewer than half the calories and one-fourth of the saturated fat.

- **3 cups unsalted gluten-free chicken stock**
- **1¾ cups broccoli florets, coarsely chopped (about 8 ounces)**
- **1 cup diced yellow onion**
- **½ cup chopped carrot**
- **⅜ teaspoon salt**
- **¼ teaspoon freshly ground black pepper**
- **2 garlic cloves, minced**
- **4 ounces reduced-fat extra-sharp cheddar cheese, shredded and divided (about 1 cup)**
- **¾ cup half-and-half**
- **¼ cup fresh flat-leaf parsley leaves**

1. Combine first 7 ingredients in a large saucepan; bring to a boil. Reduce heat, and simmer 10 minutes or until broccoli is tender. Pour soup into a blender. Remove center piece of blender lid (to allow steam to escape); secure lid on blender. Place a clean towel over opening in blender lid (to avoid splatters). Blend until smooth. Return soup to pan. Stir in 2 ounces cheese and half-and-half. Top with remaining cheese and parsley.

YIELD | SERVES 4 (SERVING SIZE: ABOUT 1 CUP SOUP AND 2 TABLESPOONS CHEESE)

CALORIES 160; FAT 7.4g (sat 4.5g, mono 2.1g, poly 0.3g); PROTEIN 14g; CARB 11g; FIBER 2g; CHOL 23mg; IRON 1mg; SODIUM 532mg; CALC 213mg

Black Bean Soup

- **1** cup dried black beans
- **2½** tablespoons extra-virgin olive oil, divided
- **¾** cup chopped onion
- **7** garlic cloves, minced and divided
- **2½** cups gluten-free, fat-free, lower-sodium chicken broth
- **2** cups water
- **¼** cup unsalted tomato paste
- **1** teaspoon dried oregano
- **¾** teaspoon salt
- **¾** teaspoon ground cumin
- **¼** teaspoon ground red pepper
- **1** (4-ounce) can chopped green chiles
- **1** cup fresh cilantro leaves
- **½** jalapeño pepper, seeded
- **¼** cup Mexican crema
- **3** hard-cooked large eggs, peeled and finely chopped

1. Sort and wash beans, and place in a large Dutch oven. Cover with water; cover and let stand 8 hours. Drain beans.

2. Heat 1½ teaspoons oil in a Dutch oven over medium heat. Add onion; cook 4 minutes, stirring often. Add 5 garlic cloves; cook 1 minute. Increase heat to medium-high. Add beans, broth, and next 7 ingredients (through chiles); bring to a boil. Cover, reduce heat, and simmer 1 hour or until beans are tender. Let stand 10 minutes.

3. Place half of bean mixture in a blender. Remove center piece of blender lid (to allow steam to escape); secure blender lid on blender. Place a clean towel over opening in blender lid (to avoid splatters). Blend until smooth. Pour into a large bowl. Repeat procedure with remaining mixture. Return soup to pan; cook 5 minutes, stirring often.

4. Finely chop 1 cup cilantro and jalapeño. Combine 2 tablespoons oil, 2 garlic cloves, cilantro, jalapeño, and crema. Ladle 1¼ cups soup into each of 4 bowls; top each with 2 tablespoons crema mixture. Sprinkle soup with eggs.

YIELD | SERVES 4

CALORIES 369; FAT 18.4g (sat 5.8g, mono 7.8g, poly 1.8g); PROTEIN 18g; CARB 35g; FIBER 12g; CHOL 173mg; IRON 5mg; SODIUM 829mg; CALC 114mg

NO MATTER WHAT DIET YOU ARE ON, KEEPING DINNER FRESH CAN BE CHALLENGING. This chapter offers an array of healthy meals that will provide something tasty for everyone around your dinner table—even if they aren't eating gluten free.

Salsa Flounder

Serve this dish with rice or corn tortillas.

- 1 tablespoon olive oil
- 4 (6-ounce) flounder fillets
- ½ teaspoon salt-free Cajun/Creole seasoning
- ½ cup thinly sliced shallots (about 2 shallots)
- 1 tablespoon butter, melted
- 2 garlic cloves, thinly sliced
- ¾ cup fresh salsa
- ¼ teaspoon freshly ground black pepper
- 1 tablespoon coarsely chopped cilantro
- 4 lime wedges

1. Place oven rack in middle of oven. Preheat broiler.

2. Drizzle oil in a roasting pan. Pat fish dry with paper towels; arrange fish in pan. Sprinkle fish with Cajun seasoning. Sprinkle shallots, butter, and garlic around pan. Pour salsa into pan around fish. Broil 10 minutes or until fish flakes easily when tested with a fork or until desired degree of doneness, basting frequently. Arrange fish on a platter; sprinkle with pepper. Stir cilantro into pan sauce; drizzle sauce over fish. Serve with lime wedges.

YIELD | SERVES 4 (SERVING SIZE: 1 FILLET, ABOUT 2 TABLESPOONS SAUCE, AND 1 LIME WEDGE)

CALORIES 189; FAT 9.1g (sat 2.9g, mono 4g, poly 1g); PROTEIN 19g; CARB 6g; FIBER 1g; CHOL 73mg; IRON 1mg; SODIUM 567mg; CALC 41mg

Cedar Plank Salmon with Tomato Salsa

1   (18-inch) cedar plank
1   poblano chile, seeded and halved
1   jalapeño pepper, seeded and halved
1   small red onion, cut into ½-inch-thick slices
Cooking spray
2   cups chopped seeded heirloom tomato
3   tablespoons chopped fresh cilantro
½   teaspoon kosher salt, divided
½   teaspoon freshly ground black pepper, divided
1   diced peeled avocado
1   lime, divided
4   (6-ounce) skinless salmon fillets

1. Soak plank in water 25 minutes.
2. Preheat grill to medium-high heat.
3. Place poblano, jalapeño, and onion on grill rack coated with cooking spray; grill 10 minutes, turning occasionally. Remove from grill; cool. Coarsely chop poblano and onion; finely chop jalapeño. Combine peppers, onion, tomato, cilantro, ¼ teaspoon salt, ¼ teaspoon pepper, avocado, and juice from half of lime.
4. Sprinkle fish with ¼ teaspoon salt and ¼ teaspoon black pepper. Place plank on grill rack; grill 3 minutes or until lightly charred. Turn plank over; place fish on charred side. Cover; grill 8 minutes or until desired degree of doneness. Cut remaining lime half into 4 wedges. Top each fillet with ½ cup tomato salsa. Serve with lime wedges.

YIELD | SERVES 4

CALORIES 386; FAT 20.7g (sat 4.2g, mono 10.6g, poly 4.2g); PROTEIN 38g; CARB 12g; FIBER 6g; CHOL 87mg; IRON 1mg; SODIUM 330mg; CALC 48mg

Saffron Rice with Tilapia and Shrimp

8 ounces unpeeled large shrimp
3⅓ cups gluten-free unsalted chicken stock
⅔ cup water
⅛ teaspoon saffron threads, crushed
1 cup chopped ripe tomato
1 cup chopped onion
1⅛ teaspoons salt, divided
½ teaspoon sugar
4 garlic cloves
3 tablespoons olive oil
1¼ cups uncooked short-grain rice
12 ounces tilapia, cut into 1-inch pieces
½ cup frozen green peas
¼ cup chopped fresh flat-leaf parsley
6 lemon wedges

1. Preheat oven to 450°.
2. Peel shrimp, reserving shells; set shrimp aside. Combine shrimp shells, chicken stock, ⅔ cup water, and saffron in a saucepan. Bring to a boil; reduce heat, and keep warm.
3. Combine tomato, onion, ½ teaspoon salt, sugar, and garlic in a food processor; process until smooth.
4. Heat a large ovenproof skillet over medium-high heat. Add oil to pan; swirl to coat. Add tomato mixture to pan; cook 6 minutes or until liquid almost evaporates, stirring occasionally. Add uncooked rice to pan; cook 3 minutes, stirring frequently. Drain stock mixture over a bowl; discard solids. Add stock mixture to pan; bring to a boil. Cook over medium heat 12 minutes or until rice is tender and liquid is absorbed (do not stir). Top with reserved shrimp, tilapia, and peas. Sprinkle with ⅝ teaspoon salt. Cover and bake at 450° for 15 minutes or until fish flakes easily when tested with a fork or until desired degree of doneness. Sprinkle with parsley; serve with lemon wedges.

YIELD | SERVES 6 (SERVING SIZE: ABOUT 1½ CUPS RICE MIXTURE AND 1 LEMON WEDGE)

CALORIES 338; FAT 8.8g (sat 1.5g, mono 5.4g, poly 1.4g); PROTEIN 24g; CARB 41g; FIBER 3g; CHOL 76mg; IRON 3mg; SODIUM 600mg; CALC 60mg

INGREDIENT TIP

Shrimp shells
This paella-inspired dish starts by infusing purchased chicken stock with shrimpy goodness. It's an easy step that makes full use of shrimp shells that would have otherwise been discarded.

Tilapia Veracruz

Spanish and Mexican flavors combine in this quick fish dish. Serve with steamed rice and sautéed spinach.

4	(4-ounce) tilapia fillets
½	teaspoon freshly ground black pepper
¼	teaspoon salt
1	tablespoon extra-virgin olive oil
1½	cups chopped onion
1	tablespoon chopped fresh oregano
4	garlic cloves, sliced
1	yellow bell pepper, thinly sliced
2	cups chopped tomato
2	ounces pimiento-stuffed green olives (about 20), halved
1	tablespoon capers, rinsed and drained
1	jalapeño pepper, thinly sliced

1. Sprinkle fish with pepper and salt. Heat a large nonstick skillet over medium-high heat. Add oil; swirl to coat. Add fish to pan; cook 3 minutes or until browned on one side. Remove fish from pan.

2. Add onion, oregano, garlic, and bell pepper to pan; sauté 4 minutes. Stir in tomato and remaining ingredients; bring to a simmer.

3. Arrange fish on top of tomato mixture, browned sides up. Cover, reduce heat to medium, and simmer 3 minutes or until fish flakes easily when tested with a fork or until desired degree of doneness.

YIELD | SERVES 4 (SERVING SIZE: 1 FILLET AND ½ CUP SAUCE)

CALORIES 211; FAT 7.2g (sat 1.2g, mono 4.1g, poly 1.4g); PROTEIN 25g; CARB 14g; FIBER 3g; CHOL 57mg; IRON 1mg; SODIUM 532mg; CALC 49mg

Sautéed Tilapia Tacos with Grilled Peppers and Onion

Slice the onion just before placing it on the grill. If given time to set, the onion rings will begin to separate and will not have good grill marks.

2	(½-inch-thick) slices white onion
1	(8-ounce) package mini sweet bell peppers
	Cooking spray
¾	teaspoon salt, divided
½	teaspoon freshly ground black pepper, divided
4	(5-ounce) tilapia fillets
8	(6-inch) corn tortillas
8	lime wedges (optional)

1. Preheat grill to high heat.

2. Arrange onion slices and bell peppers on a grill rack coated with cooking spray. Grill onions for 12 minutes, turning after 6 minutes. Grill bell peppers 12 minutes, turning occasionally. Remove onions and bell peppers from grill, and let stand for 5 minutes. Slice onion rings in half. Thinly slice bell peppers; discard stems and seeds. Combine onion, bell peppers, ¼ teaspoon salt, and ⅛ teaspoon black pepper in a small bowl.

3. Sprinkle fish evenly with ½ teaspoon salt and ⅜ teaspoon black pepper. Heat a large non-stick skillet over medium-high heat. Coat pan with cooking spray. Add fish to pan, and cook for 3 minutes on each side or until fish flakes easily when tested with a fork or until desired degree of doneness.

4. Warm tortillas according to package directions. Divide fish, onion mixture, and jalapeño slices evenly among tortillas. Serve with lime wedges, if desired.

YIELD | SERVES 4 (SERVING SIZE: 2 TACOS)

CALORIES 292; FAT 4.4g (sat 1.2g, mono 1.2g, poly 1.3g); PROTEIN 33g; CARB 32g; FIBER 5g; CHOL 71mg; IRON 2mg; SODIUM 526mg; CALC 120mg

Seared Scallops with Snap Peas and Pancetta

Sautéed snap peas, pancetta, and shallots make a speedy but sophisticated accompaniment to seared scallops.

- 3 teaspoons canola oil, divided
- 12 ounces sugar snap peas, trimmed and diagonally sliced
- ¼ teaspoon kosher salt, divided
- ¼ teaspoon black pepper, divided
- 1½ ounces diced pancetta (such as Boar's Head)
- 2 large shallots, sliced
- 1½ pounds large sea scallops
- 4 lemon wedges

1. Heat a large cast-iron skillet over medium-high heat. Add 1 teaspoon oil; swirl to coat. Add peas, ⅛ teaspoon salt, and ⅛ teaspoon pepper; sauté 2 minutes. Place peas in a bowl. Heat pan over medium heat. Add pancetta; cook 1 minute. Add shallots; cook 1 minute, stirring constantly. Add pancetta mixture to pea mixture.

2. Return pan to medium-high heat. Pat scallops dry with paper towels; sprinkle with ⅛ teaspoon salt and ⅛ teaspoon pepper. Add 1 teaspoon oil to pan; swirl to coat. Add half of scallops to pan; cook 2 minutes. Turn and cook 1 minute or until desired degree of doneness. Place cooked scallops on a plate. Repeat procedure with remaining 1 teaspoon oil and remaining scallops. Serve scallops with pea mixture and lemon wedges.

YIELD | SERVES 4 (SERVING SIZE: ABOUT 5 SCALLOPS AND ¾ CUP PEA MIXTURE)

CALORIES 237; FAT 7.9g (sat 2.2g, mono 2.3g, poly 1.3g); PROTEIN 25g; CARB 15g; FIBER 3g; CHOL 48mg; IRON 3mg; SODIUM 568mg; CALC 52mg

Asian Rice with Shrimp and Snow Peas

1	cup uncooked long-grain rice
1	cup water
1	cup gluten-free, fat-free, lower-sodium chicken broth
3	tablespoons gluten-free, lower-sodium soy sauce
3	tablespoons rice vinegar
1	tablespoon dark sesame oil
2	teaspoons minced fresh garlic
1	teaspoon hot sauce
2	cups snow peas, trimmed (about 6 ounces)
1½	pounds large peeled and deveined shrimp
½	cup diagonally cut green onions
4	teaspoons slivered almonds, toasted

1. Combine long-grain rice, 1 cup water, and broth in a medium saucepan; bring to a boil. Cover, reduce heat, and simmer 20 minutes or until liquid is absorbed.

2. Combine soy sauce, vinegar, sesame oil, garlic, and hot sauce in a large bowl; stir with a whisk. Set aside.

3. Cook snow peas and shrimp in boiling water 2 minutes or until shrimp are done. Drain. Add snow peas, shrimp, green onions, and rice to soy mixture; toss well to combine. Top with almonds. Serve immediately.

YIELD | SERVES 4 (SERVING SIZE: 2 CUPS SHRIMP MIXTURE AND 1 TEASPOON ALMONDS)

CALORIES 334; FAT 7.6g (sat 1.2g, mono 1.9g; poly 3.5g); PROTEIN 39g; CARB 25g; FIBER 2g; CHOL 259mg; IRON 6mg; SODIUM 776mg; CALC 129mg

Slow-Cooker Brisket

1 (4½-pound) flat-cut brisket roast, fat cap trimmed to ⅛-inch thickness
1¼ teaspoons kosher salt, divided
½ teaspoon freshly ground black pepper
1 tablespoon canola oil
1½ teaspoons garlic powder
1 teaspoon paprika
3 medium carrots, peeled and cut into thirds
3 celery stalks, cut into thirds
Cooking spray
2 large onions, halved and vertically sliced
4 garlic cloves, chopped
1 cup gluten-free unsalted beef stock
2 tablespoons brown sugar
2 tablespoons cider vinegar
1 (15-ounce) can crushed tomatoes, undrained
5 thyme sprigs
2 bay leaves

1. Sprinkle brisket with 1 teaspoon salt and pepper. Heat a large skillet over medium-high heat. Add oil; swirl to coat. Add brisket; cook 5 minutes, turning to brown on all sides. Rub brisket with garlic powder and paprika. Arrange carrots and celery in a 6-quart electric slow cooker coated with cooking spray; top with brisket, fat cap side up.

2. Return pan to medium heat. Add onions to pan; cover and cook 10 minutes, stirring occasionally. Uncover. Stir in garlic; cook 5 minutes or until onions are tender and golden. Arrange onion mixture over brisket.

3. Combine ¼ teaspoon salt, stock, brown sugar, vinegar, and tomatoes in hot pan, stirring with a whisk to loosen browned bits. Pour tomato mixture around brisket. Place thyme and bay leaves in slow cooker, pressing into tomato mixture. Cover and cook on LOW 7 hours or until brisket is tender. Cool slightly in cooker, about 1 hour.

4. Place brisket on a cutting board. Trim fat cap; discard fat. Cut brisket across grain into thin slices. Pour sauce through a sieve over a bowl; discard carrots, celery, thyme, and bay leaves. Return onions to sauce. Serve brisket with sauce.

YIELD | SERVES 12 (SERVING SIZE: ABOUT 3 OUNCES BEEF AND ABOUT ⅔ CUP SAUCE)

CALORIES 307; **FAT** 15.1g (sat 5g, mono 7.1g, poly 0.8g); **PROTEIN** 33g; **CARB** 8g; **FIBER** 1g; **CHOL** 100mg; **IRON** 4mg; **SODIUM** 338mg; **CALC** 31mg

Cast-Iron Burgers

1 pound ground sirloin
¼ teaspoon kosher salt
1 tablespoon canola mayonnaise
1 tablespoon Dijon mustard
1 tablespoon prepared horseradish
2 teaspoons ketchup
2 applewood-smoked bacon slices, chopped
3 cups vertically sliced yellow onion
1 tablespoon finely chopped fresh chives
1 teaspoon gluten-free Worcestershire sauce
¼ teaspoon freshly ground black pepper
Cooking spray
4 (2.8-ounce) gluten-free hamburger buns, toasted
4 green leaf lettuce leaves
4 (¼-inch-thick) slices tomato

1. Divide beef into 4 portions, lightly shaping each into a ½-inch-thick patty. Sprinkle with salt. Cover and refrigerate 30 minutes.

2. Combine mayonnaise and next 3 ingredients (through ketchup) in a small bowl. Set aside.

3. Cook bacon in a large nonstick skillet over medium-low heat until crisp. Remove bacon from pan. Add onion to drippings in pan; cook 15 minutes or until golden brown. Combine bacon, onion, chives, Worcestershire sauce, and pepper in a small bowl.

4. Heat a large cast-iron skillet over medium-high heat. Coat pan with cooking spray. Add patties; cook 2 minutes on each side or until desired degree of doneness. Spread 1½ teaspoons horseradish spread on cut side of each bun half. Top bottom half of each bun with 1 lettuce leaf, 1 tomato slice, 1 patty, ¼ cup relish, and top half of bun.

YIELD | SERVES 4 (SERVING SIZE: 1 BURGER)

CALORIES 420; FAT 16.6g (sat 5.9g, mono 5.9g, poly 1.5g); PROTEIN 30g; CARB 36g; FIBER 4g; CHOL 79mg; IRON 5mg; SODIUM 814mg; CALC 126mg

Roasted Pork Tenderloin Tacos

1   **(1-pound) pork tenderloin, trimmed**
½   **teaspoon freshly ground black pepper**
¼   **teaspoon salt**
1   **tablespoon canola oil**
2   **tablespoons mojo marinade (such as Goya)**
½   **cup white wine vinegar**
3   **tablespoons water**
1½   **tablespoons sugar**
1   **cup thinly vertically sliced red onion**
8   **(6-inch) corn tortillas**
1   **jalapeño pepper, cut into 16 slices**
1   **ripe peeled avocado, cut into 16 wedges**
¼   **cup Mexican crema**

1. Preheat oven to 425°.

2. Sprinkle pork with pepper and salt. Heat a large ovenproof skillet over medium-high heat. Add oil to pan; swirl to coat. Add pork; cook 5 minutes, turning to brown on all sides. Place pan in oven. Bake at 425° for 8 minutes or until a thermometer registers 145° (slightly pink); let stand 5 minutes. Cut crosswise into 16 slices. Combine pork and mojo marinade in a medium bowl; toss to coat pork.

3. Combine vinegar, 3 tablespoons water, and sugar in a small saucepan; bring to a boil. Remove from heat; add onion. Let stand 10 minutes; drain.

4. Working with 1 tortilla at a time, toast in a pan or over the flame of a gas burner until tender and blackened in spots. Arrange 2 pork slices in center of each tortilla; top with about 2 tablespoons onion, 2 jalapeño slices, 2 avocado wedges, and 1½ teaspoons crema.

YIELD | SERVES 4 (SERVING SIZE: 2 TACOS)

CALORIES 362; **FAT** 16.9g (sat 2.1g, mono 8g, poly 2.8g); **PROTEIN** 28g; **CARB** 27g; **FIBER** 6g; **CHOL** 82mg; **IRON** 2mg; **SODIUM** 423mg; **CALC** 55mg

INGREDIENT TIP

Mexican crema

Thick and slightly tangy Mexican crema adds a cooling finish to these tacos. If you can't find it at the grocery, substitute sour cream thinned with a little lime juice.

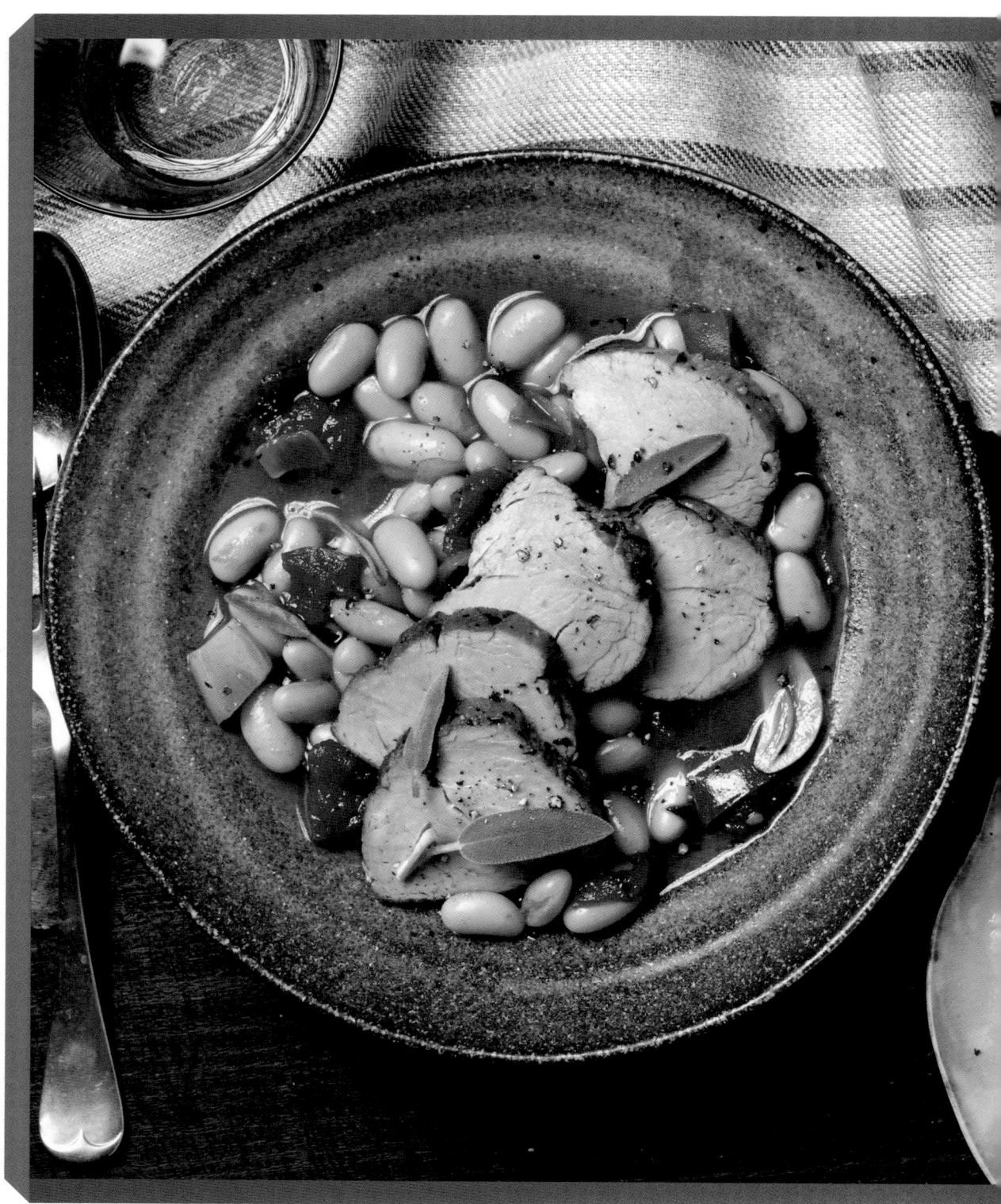

Pork Tenderloin and Cannellini Beans

1	teaspoon chopped fresh rosemary
¾	teaspoon kosher salt, divided
¾	teaspoon freshly ground black pepper, divided
½	teaspoon fennel seeds, lightly crushed
1	(1-pound) pork tenderloin, trimmed
1	tablespoon olive oil
½	cup chopped onion
4	large garlic cloves, thinly sliced
1	cup chopped tomato
1	teaspoon chopped fresh sage
1	cup gluten-free unsalted chicken stock
¼	teaspoon crushed red pepper
1	(15-ounce) can unsalted cannellini beans, rinsed and drained
2	tablespoons chopped fresh flat-leaf parsley

1. Preheat oven to 425°.

2. Combine rosemary, ½ teaspoon salt, ½ teaspoon black pepper, and fennel seeds in a small bowl. Rub spice mixture over pork.

3. Heat a large skillet over medium-high heat. Add oil; swirl to coat. Add pork; cook 9 minutes, browning on all sides. Remove pork from pan. Add onion and garlic; sauté 2 minutes. Add tomato and sage; cook 1 minute, scraping pan to loosen browned bits. Add ¼ teaspoon salt, ¼ teaspoon black pepper, stock, red pepper, and cannellini beans, and bring to a boil. Return pork to pan, and place pan in oven. Bake at 425° for 12 minutes or until a thermometer registers 140°.

4. Place pork on a cutting board; let stand 5 minutes. Heat pan over medium heat; cook bean mixture 2 minutes or until slightly thick. Sprinkle with parsley. Thinly slice pork; serve with bean mixture.

YIELD | SERVES 4 (SERVING SIZE: ABOUT 3 OUNCES PORK AND ½ CUP BEAN MIXTURE)

CALORIES 227; **FAT** 6.5g (sat 1.3g, mono 3.4g, poly 0.8g); **PROTEIN** 30g; **CARB** 13g; **FIBER** 3g; **CHOL** 74mg; **IRON** 2mg; **SODIUM** 475mg; **CALC** 51mg

Pork Tenderloin with Roasted Cherries and Shallots

- 2 tablespoons canola oil, divided
- ¾ teaspoon kosher salt, divided
- ½ teaspoon freshly ground black pepper
- ½ teaspoon ground cumin
- ⅛ teaspoon ground cinnamon
- 1 (1-pound) pork tenderloin, trimmed
- 8 ounces fresh cherries, pitted and halved
- 3 large shallots, quartered
- ¼ cup gluten-free unsalted chicken stock
- 2 tablespoons balsamic vinegar
- ½ teaspoon brown sugar
- 1 tablespoon butter
- ¼ cup coarsely chopped fresh flat-leaf parsley

1. Preheat oven to 425°.

2. Heat a large ovenproof skillet over medium-high heat. Add 1 tablespoon oil; swirl to coat. Combine ½ teaspoon salt, pepper, cumin, and cinnamon. Rub pork with spice mixture. Add pork to pan; sauté 4 minutes. Turn pork over; place pan in oven and bake at 425° for 15 minutes or until a thermometer registers 140°. Remove pork from pan; place on a cutting board (do not wipe out pan). Let pork stand 10 minutes. Cut into thin slices.

3. Add 1 tablespoon oil to pan; swirl to coat. Add cherries and shallots; sprinkle with ¼ teaspoon salt. Place pan in oven; bake at 425° for 10 minutes (do not turn cherries). Carefully remove pan from oven; place over medium-high heat. Stir in stock, vinegar, and sugar; bring to a boil. Cook 4 minutes or until liquid is syrupy. Remove from heat; stir in butter. Serve cherry mixture with pork; sprinkle with parsley.

YIELD | SERVES 4 (SERVING SIZE: 3 OUNCES PORK AND ABOUT ⅔ CUP SAUCE)

CALORIES 270; FAT 12.5g (sat 3.2g, mono 6.1g, poly 2.5g); PROTEIN 25g; CARB 14g; FIBER 2g; CHOL 81mg; IRON 2mg; SODIUM 458mg; CALC 27mg

Citrus-Herb Chicken

Citrus zest perfumes the chicken while it marinates. A fresh salsa of citrus segments and herbs doubles down on fruit flavor.

2	large limes
1	large ruby red grapefruit
1	large tangerine
1	large navel orange
¼	cup extra-virgin olive oil, divided
1	tablespoon minced garlic
1	tablespoon minced serrano chile
1	(3½-pound) whole chicken
¾	teaspoon kosher salt, divided
⅜	teaspoon freshly ground black pepper, divided
1	cup vertically sliced red onion
¼	cup chopped fresh mint
2	tablespoons chopped fresh cilantro

1. Grate 1 teaspoon rind and squeeze 5 tablespoons juice from limes. Place rind and 4 tablespoons juice in a medium bowl; place 1 tablespoon juice in a separate medium bowl. Grate 1 teaspoon grapefruit rind; section grapefruit. Grate 1 teaspoon tangerine rind; section tangerine. Grate 1 teaspoon orange rind; section orange. Add citrus sections to 1 tablespoon lime juice in bowl; set aside. Add rinds to lime rind mixture. Add 2 tablespoons oil, garlic, and chile to rind mixture; stir with a whisk.

2. Place chicken, breast side down, on a cutting board. Using poultry shears, cut along both sides of backbone, and open chicken like a book. Turn chicken breast side up; using the heel of your hand, press firmly against the breastbone until it cracks. Lift wing tips up and over back; tuck under chicken. Discard backbone and skin. Place chicken on a rimmed baking sheet. Spread citrus rind mixture over chicken. Cover and refrigerate at least 4 hours.

3. Position oven rack in lower third of oven. Preheat broiler.

4. Sprinkle chicken with ½ teaspoon salt and ¼ teaspoon black pepper. Broil chicken, breast side down, 20 minutes. Turn chicken over; broil an additional 20 minutes or until done, turning pan occasionally. Let stand 10 minutes.

5. Combine reserved citrus section mixture, 2 tablespoons oil, ¼ teaspoon salt, ⅛ teaspoon pepper, red onion, mint, and cilantro; toss to combine.

YIELD | SERVES 4 (SERVING SIZE: ¼ OF CHICKEN AND ½ CUP SALSA)

CALORIES 369; FAT 17.6g (sat 2.9g, mono 11.1g, poly 2.4g); PROTEIN 31g; CARB 24g; FIBER 7g; CHOL 92mg; IRON 3mg; SODIUM 473mg; CALC 76mg

Chicken with Turnips and Pomegranate Sauce

3	cups gluten-free unsalted chicken stock, divided
1	cup uncooked wild rice
1	tablespoon chopped fresh thyme leaves
1¼	teaspoons black pepper, divided
¾	teaspoon kosher salt, divided
1	cup pomegranate juice
½	cup pomegranate arils
2	large turnips, peeled and cut into ¼-inch slices
2	tablespoons olive oil, divided
4	(6-ounce) skinless, boneless chicken breast halves

1. Preheat oven to 400°.

2. Combine 2 cups stock, rice, and thyme in a medium saucepan. Bring to a boil. Cover, reduce heat, and simmer 50 minutes. Drain. Stir in ½ teaspoon pepper and ¼ teaspoon salt.

3. Combine 1 cup stock and juice in a saucepan. Bring to a boil; reduce heat, and cook 20 minutes or until mixture is reduced to ⅓ cup. Remove from heat; stir in arils.

4. Combine turnips, ½ teaspoon pepper, ¼ teaspoon salt, and 1 tablespoon oil in a bowl; toss to coat. Arrange turnip mixture on a baking sheet. Bake at 400° for 20 minutes or until browned and tender, turning once.

5. Sprinkle ¼ teaspoon salt and ¼ teaspoon pepper over chicken. Heat a large ovenproof skillet over medium-high heat. Add 1 tablespoon oil to pan; swirl to coat. Add chicken; cook 4 minutes. Turn chicken, and place pan in oven. Bake at 400° for 8 minutes or until chicken is done.

6. Spoon about ½ cup rice onto each of 4 plates. Top with about ⅓ cup turnips and 1 chicken breast half. Drizzle each with about 4 teaspoons pomegranate sauce.

YIELD | SERVES 4

CALORIES 489; FAT 11.7g (sat 2g, mono 6.3g, poly 1.7g); PROTEIN 45g; CARB 51g; FIBER 4g; CHOL 109mg; IRON 2mg; SODIUM 678mg; CALC 68mg

Shredded Chicken Tacos with Tomatoes and Grilled Corn

2   ears shucked corn
1   (12-ounce) package baby heirloom tomatoes
½   teaspoon freshly ground black pepper
¼   teaspoon salt
8   (6-inch) corn tortillas
2   cups shredded skinless, boneless rotisserie chicken breast
1   peeled avocado, cut into 16 slices
8   lime wedges (optional)

1. Preheat broiler.
2. Place corn on a jelly-roll pan; broil 18 minutes or until charred on all sides, rotating every 6 minutes. Cut kernels from corn; place kernels in a medium bowl. Cut tomatoes into quarters. Add tomatoes to corn, and sprinkle corn mixture with black pepper and salt.
3. Heat tortillas according to package directions. Divide chicken evenly among tortillas; top each taco with ¼ cup corn mixture and 2 avocado slices. Serve with lime wedges, if desired.

YIELD | SERVES 4 (SERVING SIZE: 2 TACOS)

CALORIES 420; **FAT** 13.5g (sat 2.3g, mono 7.1g, poly 2.4g); **PROTEIN** 39g; **CARB** 41g; **FIBER** 8g; **CHOL** 101mg; **IRON** 2mg; **SODIUM** 554mg; **CALC** 123mg

Greek-Style Chicken Breasts

Cooking spray

4 (6-ounce) skinless, boneless chicken breast halves

¼ teaspoon kosher salt

¼ teaspoon freshly ground black pepper

1½ tablespoons olive oil

1¾ cups vertically sliced onion

1 tablespoon minced garlic

1 ounce chopped pitted kalamata olives (about 14)

1 medium tomato, halved and sliced

¼ cup chopped fresh flat-leaf parsley

2 teaspoons chopped fresh oregano

2 teaspoons fresh lemon juice

1 ounce feta cheese, crumbled (about ¼ cup)

1. Heat a grill pan over medium-high heat. Coat pan with cooking spray. Sprinkle chicken with salt and pepper. Add chicken to pan; cook 6 minutes on each side or until done.

2. Heat a large skillet over medium-high heat. Add oil to pan; swirl to coat. Add onion and garlic; sauté 4 minutes. Add olives and tomato; cook 3 minutes or until tomato begins to break down, stirring occasionally. Remove pan from heat; stir in parsley, oregano, and juice. Top chicken with tomato and olive mixture; sprinkle feta over chicken.

YIELD | SERVES 4 (SERVING SIZE: 1 CHICKEN BREAST HALF, ABOUT ⅓ CUP TOMATO MIXTURE, AND ABOUT 1 TABLESPOON FETA)

CALORIES 311; FAT 13.2g (sat 3g, mono 6.8g, poly 1.5g); PROTEIN 38g; CARB 8g; FIBER 2g; CHOL 115mg; IRON 1mg; SODIUM 518mg; CALC 74mg

Chicken Verde Enchiladas

How do you shred chicken superfast? Insert two forks into the meat while it's still warm. Then pull apart to shred.

- ¾ **cup chopped onion**
- ¾ **cup gluten-free unsalted chicken stock**
- ½ **cup salsa verde**
- ⅓ **cup finely chopped cilantro stems**
- 2 **tablespoons sliced pickled jalapeño pepper**
- 5 **teaspoons gluten-free all-purpose flour**
- ½ **teaspoon ground cumin**
- 2 **garlic cloves, thinly sliced**
- 8 **ounces shredded skinless, boneless rotisserie chicken breast (about 2 cups)**
- ¾ **cup chopped tomato**
- 3 **tablespoons reduced-fat sour cream**
- 1 **ripe peeled avocado, coarsely mashed**
- 8 **(6-inch) corn tortillas**
- 4 **ounces reduced-fat sharp cheddar cheese, shaved (about 1 cup)**
- 2 **tablespoons cilantro leaves**

1. Position oven rack in lower third of oven, and preheat broiler.

2. Combine first 8 ingredients in a medium saucepan, stirring with a whisk. Bring to a boil; reduce heat, and simmer 4 minutes. Stir in chicken; cook 1 minute or until heated. Remove from heat. Stir in tomato, sour cream, and avocado.

3. Stack tortillas; wrap stack in damp paper towels, and microwave at HIGH 45 seconds. Spoon 1 cup chicken mixture into an 11 x 7–inch glass or ceramic baking dish. Spoon ⅓ cup chicken mixture in center of each tortilla; roll up. Arrange tortillas, seam sides down, in baking dish. Top with cheese. Broil 3 minutes or until cheese melts. Sprinkle with cilantro leaves.

YIELD | SERVES 4 (SERVING SIZE: 2 ENCHILADAS)

CALORIES 400; FAT 18g (sat 6.5g, mono 7.9g, poly 2g); PROTEIN 29g; CARB 33g; FIBER 7g; CHOL 75mg; IRON 1mg; SODIUM 620mg; CALC 267mg

Braised Chicken with Honey-Lemon Leeks

Lemon is a bright partner for the caramelized leeks, which cook twice: They are sautéed, then roasted to meld with the honey and lemon.

- **4 teaspoons olive oil, divided**
- **8 bone-in, skinless chicken thighs (about 2 pounds)**
- **¾ teaspoon kosher salt, divided**
- **½ teaspoon freshly ground black pepper**
- **1 tablespoon grated lemon rind**
- **4 cups thinly sliced leek (about 3 large)**
- **3 tablespoons fresh lemon juice**
- **2 teaspoons honey**
- **2 tablespoons chopped fresh parsley or chives (optional)**

1. Preheat oven to 400°.

2. Heat a large ovenproof skillet over medium heat. Add 2 teaspoons oil to pan; swirl to coat. Sprinkle chicken with ½ teaspoon salt and pepper. Massage lemon rind into chicken. Place chicken in pan; cook 4 minutes on each side or until browned. Remove chicken from pan; keep warm.

3. Add 2 teaspoons oil to pan; swirl to coat. Add leek and ¼ teaspoon salt; cook 15 minutes or until leek begins to brown, scraping pan to loosen browned bits. Remove pan from heat; stir in juice and honey. Return chicken to pan. Mound leeks on top of chicken thighs. Bake chicken at 400° for 15 minutes or until a thermometer registers 165°. Top with fresh parsley or chives, if desired.

YIELD | SERVES 4 (SERVING SIZE: 2 THIGHS AND ABOUT ¼ CUP LEEK MIXTURE)

CALORIES 339; FAT 15.6g (sat 3.6g, mono 7.7g, poly 2.8g); PROTEIN 33g; CARB 17g; FIBER 2g; CHOL 175mg; IRON 4mg; SODIUM 492mg; CALC 72mg

Grilled Chicken Thighs with Cilantro-Mint Chutney

3   **tablespoons grated fresh onion**
½   **teaspoon ground red pepper**
10   **garlic cloves, minced**
2½ **tablespoons canola oil, divided**
2   **teaspoons ground cumin, divided**
4   **(6-ounce) bone-in chicken thighs**
½   **teaspoon kosher salt, divided**
Cooking spray
1   **cup cilantro leaves**
½   **cup mint leaves**
⅓   **cup chopped green onions**
2   **teaspoons chopped seeded jalapeño pepper**

1. Combine first 3 ingredients in a large zip-top plastic bag; stir in 2 tablespoons oil and 1¾ teaspoons cumin. Add chicken to bag, seal, and massage marinade into chicken. Marinate in refrigerator 2 hours.
2. Preheat grill to medium-high heat.
3. Remove chicken from bag. Sprinkle chicken with ¼ teaspoon salt. Place on grill rack coated with cooking spray; grill 8 minutes on each side.
4. Place cilantro, mint, green onions, and jalapeño in a food processor; process until combined. Add 1½ teaspoons oil, ¼ teaspoon cumin, and ¼ teaspoon salt; process until smooth. Serve chicken topped with chutney.

YIELD | SERVES 4 (SERVING SIZE: 1 THIGH AND ABOUT 1½ TABLESPOONS CHUTNEY)

CALORIES 331; FAT 24g (sat 4.8g, mono 11.8g, poly 5.5g); PROTEIN 24g; CARB 5g; FIBER 1g; CHOL 135mg; IRON 2mg; SODIUM 332mg; CALC 46mg

Dijon-Herb Chicken Thighs

2	tablespoons chopped fresh flat-leaf parsley
2	tablespoons chopped fresh chives
2	tablespoons olive oil
2	teaspoons Dijon mustard
2	garlic cloves, minced
4	(6-ounce) bone-in chicken thighs (about 1½ pounds), skinned
½	teaspoon kosher salt
½	teaspoon freshly ground black pepper
	Cooking spray

1. Preheat oven to 450°.

2. Combine parsley, chives, olive oil, Dijon mustard, and garlic in a small bowl, stirring well with a whisk. Rub herb mixture over meaty side of chicken thighs; sprinkle with salt and pepper.

3. Arrange chicken on a baking sheet or jelly-roll pan coated with cooking spray. Bake at 450° for 25 minutes or until done.

4. Preheat broiler (do not remove pan from oven). Broil chicken 3 minutes or until browned.

YIELD | SERVES 4 (SERVING SIZE: 1 THIGH)

CALORIES 270; FAT 13.9g (sat 2.7g, mono 7.4g, poly 2.3g); PROTEIN 33g; CARB 1g; FIBER 0g; CHOL 162mg; IRON 2mg; SODIUM 453mg; CALC 23mg

Five-Bean Chili

Serving this chili the next day lets flavors meld—if the beans soak up a lot of liquid overnight, you can add more vegetable broth or even water to thin it out.

1	tablespoon canola oil
2	cups chopped onion
1	cup chopped carrot
2	tablespoons unsalted tomato paste
2	tablespoons minced fresh garlic
1½	teaspoons dried oregano
1½	teaspoons chili powder
1	teaspoon kosher salt
½	teaspoon Spanish smoked paprika
4	cups stemmed and torn kale
3	cups gluten-free organic vegetable broth
2	red bell peppers, chopped
1	jalapeño pepper, seeded and chopped
1	(16-ounce) can unsalted pinto beans, rinsed and drained
1	(15.8-ounce) can unsalted Great Northern beans, rinsed and drained
1	(15.5-ounce) can unsalted chickpeas (garbanzo beans), rinsed and drained
1	(15-ounce) can unsalted black beans, rinsed and drained
1	(15-ounce) can unsalted kidney beans, rinsed and drained
1	(14.5-ounce) can unsalted diced tomatoes, undrained

1. Heat a large Dutch oven over medium heat. Add oil; swirl to coat. Add onion and carrot; sauté 10 minutes or until tender. Stir in tomato paste and next 5 ingredients (through paprika); cook 2 minutes, stirring constantly. Add kale and remaining ingredients. Cover and simmer 45 minutes.

YIELD | SERVES 8 (SERVING SIZE: ABOUT 1½ CUPS)

CALORIES 221; FAT 2.8g (sat 0.2g, mono 1.2g, poly 0.7g); PROTEIN 11g; CARB 39g; FIBER 12g; CHOL 0mg; IRON 3mg; SODIUM 520mg; CALC 153mg

Stuffed Poblanos

8   large poblano peppers
4   dried ancho chiles
2   tablespoons canola oil
3   cups chopped onion
10   garlic cloves, minced
12   ounces ground sirloin
1   teaspoon kosher salt, divided
1   teaspoon black pepper
4   ounces ⅓-less-fat cream cheese, softened (about ½ cup)
1½   cups precooked brown rice (such as Uncle Ben's Ready Rice)
6   ounces queso fresco, crumbled and divided (about 1½ cups)
¼   cup fresh lime juice
1   tablespoon ground cumin
2   teaspoons sugar
2   (14.5-ounce) cans unsalted diced tomatoes, undrained
Cooking spray
¼   cup cilantro leaves

1. Preheat broiler.

2. Place poblanos on a foil-lined baking sheet; broil 3 inches from heat 12 minutes or until blackened, turning after 6 minutes. Place in a paper bag; fold to close tightly. Let stand 15 minutes. Peel and discard skins. Cut a lengthwise slit in each pepper; discard seeds and membranes. Set aside.

3. Place ancho chiles in a bowl. Cover with boiling water; let stand 10 minutes. Drain.

4. Reduce oven temperature to 400°.

5. Heat a large skillet over medium heat. Add oil to pan; swirl. Add onion and garlic; cook 4 minutes or until crisp-tender. Reserve half of onion mixture. Add beef, ½ teaspoon salt, and black pepper; cook 8 minutes or until beef is done. Remove from heat. Add cream cheese, stirring until well combined. Stir in rice and half of queso fresco.

6. Place ancho chiles, reserved onion mixture, juice, cumin, sugar, tomatoes, and ½ teaspoon salt in a blender; process until smooth. Pour 1 cup sauce into each of 2 (8-inch) square glass or ceramic baking dishes coated with cooking spray. Open each poblano chile; flatten slightly. Divide beef mixture among chiles (they will be full). Arrange 4 chiles in each dish; top with remaining sauce and queso. Bake at 400° for 20 minutes or until bubbly. Sprinkle with cilantro.

YIELD | SERVES 8 (SERVING SIZE: 1 STUFFED CHILE AND ABOUT ⅔ CUP SAUCE)

CALORIES 334; FAT 14.8g (sat 5.2g, mono 5.5g, poly 1.8g); PROTEIN 18g; CARB 35g; FIBER 7g; CHOL 45mg; IRON 4mg; SODIUM 369mg; CALC 148mg

INGREDIENT TIP

Too hot? Poblano peppers range in heat level from quite spicy to rather mild, and there's no way to know what you're getting until you take a bite. If your peppers are too hot, cool off with a dollop of sour cream.

Sausage Pizza

- 2 teaspoons granulated sugar
- 1 package dry yeast (about 2¼ teaspoons)
- ½ cup warm water (100° to 110°)
- 3.65 ounces white rice flour (about ¾ cup)
- 1.4 ounces sweet white sorghum flour (about ⅓ cup)
- 1.4 ounces tapioca flour (about ⅓ cup)
- 1.7 ounces potato starch (about ⅓ cup)
- 0.9 ounce flaxseed meal (about ¼ cup)
- 1 teaspoon xanthan gum
- ¼ teaspoon salt
- 1 tablespoon olive oil
- 2 large egg whites
- 1 large egg
- Cooking spray
- 4 ounces turkey Italian sausage (1 link)
- ½ cup gluten-free, lower-sodium marinara sauce
- 4 ounces part-skim mozzarella cheese, shredded (about 1 cup)
- 2 tablespoons chopped ripe olives

1. Dissolve sugar and yeast in ½ cup warm water in a bowl; let stand 5 minutes.

2. Weigh or lightly spoon flours, potato starch, and flaxseed meal into dry measuring cups; level with a knife. Combine flours, potato starch, flaxseed meal, xanthan gum, and salt in a bowl; beat with a mixer at medium speed until blended. Add yeast mixture, oil, egg whites, and egg; beat at low speed until combined. Increase speed to medium; beat 2 minutes.

3. Spoon dough onto an 11 x 17–inch baking sheet coated with cooking spray and lined with parchment paper. Lightly coat hands with cooking spray; press dough into an 11 x 12–inch rectangle. Cover with plastic wrap coated with cooking spray, and let rise in a warm place (85°), free from drafts, 30 minutes.

4. Preheat oven to 400°.

5. Remove plastic wrap. Bake at 400° for 14 minutes or until bottom is crisp. Cool completely. Increase oven temperature to 425°.

6. Remove casing from sausage. Heat a large skillet over medium-high heat. Add sausage; cook 3 minutes. Spread marinara over crust, leaving a ½-inch border; top with sausage, cheese, and olives. Bake at 425° for 12 minutes or until golden.

YIELD | SERVES 6 (SERVING SIZE: 1 RECTANGLE)

CALORIES 309; FAT 11.8g (sat 3.6g, mono 4.7g, poly 2.2g); PROTEIN 15g; CARB 37g; FIBER 3.5g; CHOL 63mg; IRON 1.3mg; SODIUM 564mg; CALC 19mg

Vegetarian Lasagna

9   uncooked gluten-free lasagna noodles
1   teaspoon olive oil
7   cups sliced mushrooms
3   cups sliced shiitake mushroom caps
½   teaspoon ground nutmeg
3   garlic cloves, minced
6   tablespoons grated fresh Parmesan cheese, divided
1   teaspoon dried Italian seasoning
1   teaspoon freshly ground black pepper
3   large egg whites
2   (15-ounce) cartons part-skim ricotta cheese
2   (10-ounce) packages frozen chopped spinach, thawed, drained, and squeezed dry
1   (25.5-ounce) jar gluten-free marinara sauce
   Cooking spray
12   ounces shredded part-skim mozzarella cheese, divided (about 3 cups)

1. Cook lasagna noodles according to package directions, omitting salt and fat. Drain; set aside.

2. Heat oil in a nonstick skillet over medium heat. Add mushrooms; sauté 3 minutes. Add nutmeg and garlic; sauté 5 minutes. Set aside.

3. Combine ¼ cup Parmesan cheese, Italian seasoning, pepper, egg whites, ricotta, and spinach; set aside.

4. Preheat oven to 375°.

5. Spread ½ cup marinara sauce in bottom of a 13 x 9–inch glass or ceramic baking dish coated with cooking spray. Arrange 3 lasagna noodles over sauce; top with half of ricotta cheese mixture, half of mushroom mixture, 1½ cups sauce, and 1 cup mozzarella cheese. Repeat layers, ending with noodles. Spread ½ cup sauce over noodles.

6. Cover and bake at 375° for 40 minutes. Uncover; sprinkle with 1 cup mozzarella cheese and 2 tablespoons Parmesan cheese; bake 10 minutes. Let stand 10 minutes before serving.

YIELD | SERVES 9

CALORIES 430; FAT 17g (sat 10.1g, mono 2.8g, poly 0.5g); PROTEIN 30g; CARB 39g; FIBER 4g; CHOL 52mg; IRON 3mg; SODIUM 741mg; CALC 661mg

Three-Cheese Baked Penne

Since gluten-free pasta can clump and stick together if it stands for a while, be sure to cook it al dente (since it'll cook a bit more while it bakes), and have it ready just in time to toss with the sauce.

2	teaspoons olive oil
1½	cups finely chopped onion (about 1 medium)
1	(12-ounce) package gluten-free brown rice penne
4	cups 1% low-fat milk or dairy-free alternative, divided
¼	cup cornstarch
¾	teaspoon salt
½	teaspoon freshly ground black pepper
½	teaspoon grated whole nutmeg
4	ounces reduced-fat sharp cheddar cheese, shredded (about 1 cup)
4	ounces shredded part-skim mozzarella cheese (about 1 cup)
	Cooking spray
2	ounces grated fresh Parmesan cheese (about ½ cup)
¼	cup gluten-free panko (Japanese breadcrumbs)

1. Preheat oven to 375°.

2. Heat oil in a medium Dutch oven over medium heat. Add onion; cook 5 minutes or until tender, stirring often.

3. While onion cooks, cook pasta according to package directions, omitting salt and fat. Drain.

4. Combine ½ cup milk and cornstarch in a small bowl. Add 3½ cups milk to onion; bring to a boil. Gradually stir in cornstarch mixture. Cook 2 minutes or until sauce thickens, stirring constantly. Remove from heat, and stir in salt, pepper, and nutmeg. Add cheddar and mozzarella cheeses, stirring with a whisk until cheeses melt. Stir in pasta. Pour pasta mixture into 6 (2-cup) gratin dishes or ramekins coated with cooking spray. Combine Parmesan cheese and panko; sprinkle over pasta mixture. Bake at 375° for 30 minutes or until sauce is bubbly and top is brown.

YIELD | SERVES 6 (SERVING SIZE: ABOUT 1¼ CUPS)

CALORIES 493; FAT 14.5g (sat 7.7g, mono 3.4g, poly 0.5g); PROTEIN 23g; CARB 67g; FIBER 2g; CHOL 40mg; IRON 4mg; SODIUM 308mg; CALC 767mg

Tomato-Basil Pasta with Asiago

- 2 cups (6 ounces) uncooked gluten-free rice penne
- ¾ cup canned unsalted navy beans, rinsed and drained
- 2 tablespoons extra-virgin olive oil
- 1 cup grape tomatoes, halved
- ¼ cup finely chopped green onions
- ½ teaspoon minced fresh rosemary
- 12 pitted kalamata olives, coarsely chopped
- 2 garlic cloves, minced
- 2 cups fresh baby spinach, coarsely chopped
- 3 ounces grated Asiago cheese (about ¾ cup)
- ¼ cup chopped fresh basil
- ½ teaspoon salt
- ½ teaspoon freshly ground black pepper

1. Cook pasta according to package directions, omitting salt and fat; add beans during last 1 minute of cooking. Drain pasta and beans, reserving ¼ cup pasta water. Place pasta, beans, and reserved pasta water in a large shallow pasta bowl.

2. While pasta cooks, heat oil in a medium nonstick skillet over medium heat. Add tomatoes; cook 2 minutes, stirring often. Stir in green onions and next 3 ingredients (through garlic); cook 2 minutes or just until tomatoes are thoroughly heated. Remove from heat.

3. Add spinach and next 4 ingredients (through pepper) to pasta mixture. Toss well. Top with tomato mixture.

YIELD | SERVES 4 (SERVING SIZE: 1⅓ CUPS)

CALORIES 394; FAT 17.4g (sat 5.2g, mono 7.7g, poly 1g); PROTEIN 11g; CARB 48g; FIBER 5g; CHOL 19mg; IRON 4mg; SODIUM 718mg; CALC 243mg

INGREDIENT TIP
Fresh rosemary
You can easily strip rosemary leaves from their tough, inedible stems by holding the top of a stem in one hand, and then pulling in the opposite direction of the way the leaves grow. You can substitute ½ teaspoon crushed dried rosemary for the fresh, if you'd like.

Pasta with Roasted Red Pepper and Cream Sauce

1	pound uncooked gluten-free seashell pasta
2	teaspoons extra-virgin olive oil
½	cup finely chopped onion
1	(12-ounce) bottle roasted red bell peppers, drained and coarsely chopped
2	teaspoons balsamic vinegar
1	cup half-and-half
1	tablespoon tomato paste
⅛	teaspoon ground red pepper
4	ounces grated fresh Parmigiano-Reggiano cheese, divided (about 1 cup)

Thinly sliced fresh basil (optional)

1. Cook pasta according to package directions, omitting salt and fat. Drain and keep warm.

2. Heat oil in a large skillet over medium heat. Add onion, and cook 8 minutes or until tender, stirring frequently. Add bell peppers; cook 2 minutes or until thoroughly heated. Increase heat to medium-high. Stir in vinegar; cook 1 minute or until liquid evaporates. Remove from heat; cool 5 minutes.

3. Place bell pepper mixture in a blender; process until smooth. Return bell pepper mixture to pan; cook over low heat until warm. Combine half-and-half and tomato paste in a small bowl, stirring with a whisk. Stir tomato mixture into bell pepper mixture, stirring with a whisk until well combined. Stir in ground red pepper.

4. Combine pasta and bell pepper mixture in a large bowl. Add ½ cup cheese, tossing to coat. Spoon 1⅓ cups pasta into each of 6 bowls; top each serving with about 1½ tablespoons cheese. Garnish with basil, if desired.

YIELD | SERVES 6

CALORIES 442; FAT 12.3g (sat 6.4g, mono 2.8g, poly 0.4g); PROTEIN 14g; CARB 67g; FIBER 0g; CHOL 32mg; IRON 5mg; SODIUM 422mg; CALC 305mg

Pasta Carbonara Florentine

- 6 center-cut bacon slices, chopped
- 1 cup finely chopped onion
- 2 tablespoons dry white wine
- 1 (6-ounce) package bagged prewashed baby spinach
- 8 ounces uncooked gluten-free spaghetti
- 2 ounces grated fresh Parmesan cheese (about ½ cup)
- ½ teaspoon salt
- ½ teaspoon freshly ground black pepper
- 1 large egg
- 1 large egg white
- 3 tablespoons chopped fresh parsley

1. Heat a large nonstick skillet over medium heat. Add bacon to pan; cook 5 minutes or until crisp, stirring frequently. Remove bacon from pan, reserving 2 teaspoons drippings in pan; set bacon aside.

2. Add onion to drippings in pan; cook 3 minutes or until tender, stirring frequently. Add wine; cook 1 minute or until liquid is reduced by half. Add spinach; cook 1 minute or until spinach wilts, stirring constantly. Remove from heat; keep warm.

3. Cook pasta according to package directions, omitting salt and fat. Drain well, reserving 1 tablespoon pasta water. Immediately add pasta and reserved pasta water to spinach mixture in pan. Add reserved bacon; stir well to combine. Place pan over low heat.

4. Combine cheese and next 4 ingredients (through egg white), stirring with a whisk. Add to pasta mixture, tossing well to coat. Cook 1 minute. Remove from heat. Sprinkle with parsley. Serve immediately.

YIELD | SERVES 4 (SERVING SIZE: 1 CUP)

CALORIES 373; **FAT** 9.8g (sat 4.3g, mono 2.5g, poly 0.5g); **PROTEIN** 16g; **CARB** 55g; **FIBER** 3g; **CHOL** 72mg; **IRON** 6mg; **SODIUM** 773mg; **CALC** 257mg

SNACKS ARE A CRUCIAL COMPONENT OF ANY DIET. Keeping healthy snacks on hand that work with your meal plan is key to keeping hunger at bay. Use these snacks and sides to hold you over between meals and round out your plate.

Roasted Garlic and Chive Dip

Serve with sweet mini bell peppers or sliced summer squash. If you can find roasted garlic cloves at the salad bar in your grocery store, sub for raw garlic and skip the 8 minutes of cooking in the skillet.

½   cup unpeeled garlic cloves
½   cup plain fat-free Greek yogurt
½   cup light sour cream
2   tablespoons minced fresh chives
⅜   teaspoon salt
Dash of freshly ground black pepper

1. Heat a large nonstick skillet over medium heat. Add garlic cloves to pan; cover and cook 8 minutes or until lightly browned and tender when pierced with a fork, stirring occasionally. Cool slightly. Squeeze garlic from skins into the bowl of a mini food processor. Discard skins. Puree garlic until smooth.
2. Combine yogurt, sour cream, chives, salt, and pepper in a medium bowl, stirring well with a whisk. Add garlic to yogurt mixture, stirring with a whisk to combine.

YIELD | SERVES 8 (SERVING SIZE: ABOUT 2 TABLESPOONS)

CALORIES 42; FAT 1.7g (sat 1g, mono 0.5g, poly 0.1g); PROTEIN 2g; CARB 5g; FIBER 0g; CHOL 5mg; IRON 0mg; SODIUM 128mg; CALC 47mg

Cheddar-Bacon-Chive Dip

5   tablespoons fat-free sour cream
1   tablespoon canola mayonnaise
3   tablespoons finely shredded cheddar cheese
2   tablespoons finely chopped chives
2   slices cooked and crumbled center-cut bacon
Dash of freshly ground black pepper
2   ounces reduced-fat kettle-cooked potato chips

1. Combine sour cream, mayonnaise, cheese, chives, bacon, and black pepper. Serve with potato chips.

YIELD | SERVES 4 (SERVING SIZE: ½ OUNCE POTATO CHIPS [ABOUT 10 CHIPS] AND ABOUT 2 TABLESPOONS DIP)

CALORIES 128; FAT 7g (sat 2g, mono 3.4g, poly 0.9g); PROTEIN 4g; CARB 13g; FIBER 1g; CHOL 11mg; IRON 0mg; SODIUM 223mg; CALC 68mg

Green Goodness Dip

This dip is a riff on the classic green goddess dressing. It's made thicker with a base of pureed peas enriched with Greek yogurt and creamy avocado. Serve it with assorted fresh vegetables.

1	cup fresh or frozen green peas, thawed
1	cup plain fat-free Greek yogurt
½	cup flat-leaf parsley leaves
3	tablespoons chopped fresh chives
2	tablespoons fresh lemon juice
1	tablespoon chopped fresh tarragon
½	teaspoon kosher salt
¼	teaspoon freshly ground black pepper
3	canned anchovy fillets, drained
½	ripe peeled avocado

1. Combine all ingredients in a food processor; process until smooth.

YIELD | SERVES 8 (SERVING SIZE: ¼ CUP)

CALORIES 54; FAT 2.1g (sat 0.3g, mono 1.3g, poly 0.3g); PROTEIN 4g; CARB 5g; FIBER 2g; CHOL 1mg; IRON 1mg; SODIUM 207mg; CALC 35mg

Mozza Fruit Skewers

1	part-skim mozzarella cheese stick		8	grapes
4	pineapple chunks		2	skewers
4	strawberry halves			

1. Cut cheese stick into 4 pieces. Thread cheese, pineapple chunks, strawberry halves, and grapes onto skewers.

YIELD | SERVES 1

CALORIES 97; FAT 1.7g (sat 1g, mono 0.2g, poly 0.1g); PROTEIN 9g; CARB 13g; FIBER 1g; CHOL 5mg; IRON 0mg; SODIUM 221mg; CALC 211mg

Edamame Crunch

For the late-night munchies, try this snack. It packs in 11 grams of protein in a half-cup serving. Try it sautéed or roasted, too.

½	cup shelled edamame	**Dash of kosher salt**
1	teaspoon toasted sesame seeds	

1. Boil shelled edamame in water to cover until crisp-tender. Sprinkle with toasted sesame seeds and a dash of kosher salt.

YIELD | SERVES 1

CALORIES 117; FAT 4g (sat 0.2g, mono 0.6g, poly 0.7g); PROTEIN 11g; CARB 10g; FIBER 1g; CHOL 0mg; IRON 2mg; SODIUM 190mg; CALC 109mg

Lemon-Parmesan Popcorn

To make sure the oil is ready for the popcorn, add a couple of kernels and wait for them to pop. Once they pop, add the remaining kernels.

2 teaspoons grated lemon rind
1 teaspoon freshly ground black pepper
¼ teaspoon kosher salt
1.5 ounces Parmigiano-Reggiano cheese, finely grated (about ⅓ cup)
2 tablespoons olive oil
½ cup unpopped popcorn kernels

1. Combine lemon rind, pepper, salt, and cheese in a small bowl.
2. Heat oil in a medium, heavy saucepan over medium-high heat. Add popcorn to oil in pan; cover and cook 2 minutes or until kernels begin to pop, shaking pan frequently. Continue cooking 1 minute, shaking pan constantly. When popping slows to a couple seconds between pops, remove pan from heat. Let stand 1 minute or until all popping stops. Pour 6 cups popcorn into a large bowl; stir in half of cheese mixture. Stir in remaining 6 cups popcorn and remaining half of cheese mixture; toss to coat. Let stand 1 minute before serving.

YIELD | SERVES 6 (SERVING SIZE: 2 CUPS)

CALORIES 128; FAT 7.2g (sat 1.9g, mono 3.9g, poly 0.6g); PROTEIN 4g; CARB 12g; FIBER 3g; CHOL 6mg; IRON 1mg; SODIUM 189mg; CALC 81mg

Pan-Charred Asparagus

Toasted walnuts lend a delightful nutty crunch to this asparagus.
It's a quick and easy side and a nice change from roasted asparagus.

Cooking spray
8   **ounces (2½-inch) pieces trimmed asparagus**
1½ **teaspoons toasted walnut oil**
2   **teaspoons lemon juice**
2   **teaspoons chopped fresh tarragon**
¼   **teaspoon kosher salt**
2   **tablespoons shaved Parmigiano-Reggiano cheese**
1   **tablespoon chopped toasted walnuts**

1. Heat a medium, heavy skillet (not nonstick) over high heat 2 minutes.

2. Coat pan with cooking spray. Immediately add asparagus pieces to pan, shaking them into a single layer; cook, without stirring, 2 minutes or until asparagus is very lightly charred. Cook asparagus 5 minutes or until crisp-tender and evenly charred, tossing occasionally.

3. Remove pan from heat. Let asparagus rest 1 minute. Add walnut oil; toss to coat asparagus pieces. Add lemon juice; toss. Turn on heat if necessary to evaporate most of liquid. Sprinkle asparagus with tarragon and salt; toss. Sprinkle with cheese and walnuts. Serve immediately.

YIELD | SERVES 4 (SERVING SIZE: ABOUT ⅔ CUP)

CALORIES 52; **FAT** 4g (sat 0.7g, mono 0.8g, poly 2.2g); **PROTEIN** 3g; **CARB** 3g; **FIBER** 1g; **CHOL** 2mg; **IRON** 1mg; **SODIUM** 160mg; **CALC** 45mg

Browned Butter and Lemon Brussels Sprouts

1½	pounds Brussels sprouts, trimmed and halved		¼	teaspoon kosher salt
¼	cup water		¼	teaspoon freshly ground black pepper
2	tablespoons unsalted butter		1	teaspoon grated lemon rind
			1	tablespoon fresh lemon juice

1. Heat a large skillet over medium-high heat. Add Brussels sprouts and ¼ cup water to pan; cover and cook 5 minutes. Add butter, salt, and pepper to pan; cook, uncovered, 2 minutes. Increase heat to high; cook 1 minute, stirring frequently. Stir in lemon rind and lemon juice.

YIELD | SERVES 6 (SERVING SIZE: ABOUT ⅔ CUP)

CALORIES 84; FAT 4.2g (sat 2.5g, mono 1g, poly 0.3g); PROTEIN 4g; CARB 10g; FIBER 4g; CHOL 10mg; IRON 2mg; SODIUM 109mg; CALC 50mg

Cabbage Slaw with Mango Vinaigrette

½	cup chopped mango		½	cup diced mango
1	tablespoon canola oil		¼	cup thinly sliced green onions
1	tablespoon fresh lime juice		3	tablespoons chopped toasted cashews
¼	teaspoon salt			
5	cups thinly sliced green cabbage			

1. Combine chopped mango, canola oil, lime juice, and salt in a mini food processor; process until smooth. Place cabbage, diced mango, and green onions in a large bowl, tossing to combine. Drizzle cabbage mixture with pureed mango mixture; toss to coat. Sprinkle with cashews.

YIELD | SERVES 6 (SERVING SIZE: ABOUT ¾ CUP)

CALORIES 79; FAT 4.5g (sat 0.6g, mono 2.7g, poly 1g); PROTEIN 2g; CARB 9g; FIBER 2g; CHOL 0mg; IRON 1mg; SODIUM 110mg; CALC 32mg

Sautéed Green Beans with Spice-Glazed Pecans

The glazed pecans can be made up to three days in advance and stored in an airtight container at room temperature. Double the recipe to have some on hand for easy snacks.

- 2 tablespoons sugar
- 1 tablespoon water
- ¼ teaspoon ground cumin
- ¼ teaspoon ground red pepper
- ¾ cup coarsely chopped pecans
- 1 teaspoon minced fresh rosemary
- ½ teaspoon kosher salt, divided
- 2 pounds green beans, trimmed
- 2 tablespoons unsalted butter
- ¼ teaspoon freshly ground black pepper

1. Preheat oven to 350°. Line a jelly-roll pan with parchment paper.

2. Bring sugar, 1 tablespoon water, cumin, and red pepper to a boil in a small saucepan over medium heat, stirring constantly until sugar dissolves. Remove pan from heat; stir in pecans, rosemary, and ¼ teaspoon salt. Spread pecan mixture in an even layer on prepared pan. Bake at 350° for 12 minutes or until fragrant and browned. Cool in pan, stirring occasionally.

3. Place green beans in a large saucepan of boiling water; cook 4 minutes. Drain and plunge green beans into ice water; drain.

4. Melt butter in a nonstick skillet over medium-high heat. Add beans; sauté 5 minutes or until heated. Sprinkle ¼ teaspoon salt and black pepper over beans; toss. Place beans on a serving platter; sprinkle with pecan mixture. Serve immediately.

YIELD | SERVES 12 (SERVING SIZE: ¾ CUP)

CALORIES 96; FAT 7g (sat 1.7g, mono 3.3g, poly 1.6g); PROTEIN 2g; CARB 8g; FIBER 3g; CHOL 5mg; IRON 1mg; SODIUM 85mg; CALC 34mg

Caprese Zucchini

Cooking spray
2 medium zucchini, sliced
½ cup diced seeded tomato
2 tablespoons chopped fresh basil
2 teaspoons olive oil
1 teaspoon red wine vinegar
¼ teaspoon kosher salt
¼ teaspoon freshly ground black pepper
1 ounce shredded part-skim mozzarella cheese (about ¼ cup)

1. Heat a grill pan over medium-high heat. Coat pan with cooking spray. Grill zucchini slices 2 minutes on each side.
2. Preheat broiler.
3. Combine tomato, basil, olive oil, vinegar, salt, and pepper. Arrange grilled zucchini on a foil-lined baking sheet; top with tomato mixture and mozzarella. Broil 2 minutes or until cheese melts.

YIELD | SERVES 4 (SERVING SIZE: 4 ZUCCHINI SLICES, 2 TABLESPOONS TOMATO MIXTURE, AND 1 TABLESPOON CHEESE)

CALORIES 64; FAT 4.2g (sat 1.2g, mono 2g, poly 0.4g); PROTEIN 3g; CARB 4g; FIBER 1g; CHOL 4mg; IRON 1mg; SODIUM 175mg; CALC 72mg

Beet–Blood Orange Salad

1½ pounds halved peeled beets
1 blood orange
2 tablespoons toasted walnut oil
2 tablespoons minced shallots
½ teaspoon Dijon mustard
¼ teaspoon freshly ground black pepper
⅛ teaspoon salt
2 cups mixed greens
⅓ cup chopped unsalted, dry-roasted pistachios
2 tablespoons goat cheese

1. Wrap beets in parchment paper. Microwave at HIGH until tender (about 7 minutes). Let stand 5 minutes. Cut into 1-inch pieces.
2. Section orange over a bowl; squeeze to juice. Place sections in a bowl. Add oil, shallots, mustard, pepper, and salt to juice; stir. Add beets, greens, and orange sections; toss. Top with pistachios and cheese.

YIELD | SERVES 4 (SERVING SIZE: ABOUT ¾ CUP)

CALORIES 229; FAT 12.3g (sat 1.7g, mono 4g, poly 5.8g); PROTEIN 6g; CARB 26g; FIBER 7g; CHOL 3mg; IRON 2mg; SODIUM 247mg; CALC 58mg

Bourbon Baked Beans

Check your beans 10 to 15 minutes ahead of time to make sure they're not drying out.

1	pound dried navy beans (about 2½ cups)
3	applewood-smoked bacon slices
1	cup finely chopped onion
5	cups water, divided
½	cup maple syrup, divided
¼	cup plus 2 tablespoons bourbon, divided
¼	cup Dijon mustard
1½	teaspoons gluten-free Worcestershire sauce
¼	teaspoon freshly ground black pepper
1	tablespoon cider vinegar
1	teaspoon salt

1. Sort and wash beans; place in a large Dutch oven. Cover with water to 2 inches above beans; cover and let stand 8 hours or overnight. Drain beans. Wipe pan dry with a paper towel.
2. Preheat oven to 350°.
3. Heat pan over medium-high heat. Add bacon to pan, and cook 4 minutes or until crisp. Remove bacon from pan, reserving 1½ tablespoons drippings in pan; crumble bacon. Add onion to drippings in pan; cook 5 minutes or until onion begins to brown, stirring frequently. Add beans, bacon, 4 cups water, ¼ cup maple syrup, ¼ cup bourbon, and next 3 ingredients (through pepper) to pan. Bring to a boil; cover and bake at 350° for 2 hours.
4. Stir in 1 cup water, ¼ cup maple syrup, and 2 tablespoons bourbon. Cover and bake 1 hour or until beans are tender and liquid is almost absorbed. Stir in vinegar and salt.

YIELD | SERVES 13 (SERVING SIZE: ½ CUP)

CALORIES 199; FAT 3.1g (sat 1.1g, mono 0.7g, poly 0.5g); PROTEIN 8g; CARB 32g; FIBER 6g; CHOL 4mg; IRON 2mg; SODIUM 307mg; CALC 66mg

Simmered Pinto Beans with Chipotle Sour Cream

Refried beans can be high in fat; instead, serve these pinto beans simmered with earthy cumin.

2	teaspoons olive oil
½	cup chopped onion
½	cup chopped red bell pepper
½	teaspoon ground cumin
2	garlic cloves, minced
½	cup gluten-free unsalted chicken stock
⅛	teaspoon kosher salt
⅛	teaspoon freshly ground black pepper
1	(15-ounce) can unsalted pinto beans, rinsed and drained
1	tablespoon lemon juice
2	tablespoons chopped fresh flat-leaf parsley
¾	cup reduced-fat sour cream
3	tablespoons low-fat buttermilk
1½	teaspoons minced chipotle chiles, canned in adobo sauce

1. Heat a saucepan over medium-high heat. Add oil; swirl to coat. Add onion, bell pepper, cumin, and garlic; sauté 2 minutes. Add stock, salt, black pepper, and beans; simmer 7 minutes. Stir in juice and parsley.
2. Combine sour cream, buttermilk, and chiles; serve with beans.

YIELD | SERVES 6 (SERVING SIZE: ABOUT ¼ CUP BEANS AND 2 TABLESPOONS CREAM)

CALORIES 128; FAT 5.4g (sat 2.6g, mono 1.1g, poly 0.2g); PROTEIN 5g; CARB 14g; FIBER 4g; CHOL 16mg; IRON 1mg; SODIUM 100mg; CALC 99mg

Lemon-Caper Parmesan Potato Salad Bites

Turn "jacket potatoes" into irresistible potato salad bites. Capers offer a twist on traditional relish; they're actually pickled flower buds and add bright, briny flavor to this appetizer.

12 small red potatoes, halved (about 1¼ pounds)
2 teaspoons olive oil
½ cup light sour cream
2 tablespoons minced fresh chives, divided
2 tablespoons butter, melted
2 tablespoons finely chopped drained capers
1½ teaspoons lemon juice
½ teaspoon kosher salt
½ teaspoon freshly ground black pepper
2 tablespoons grated Parmesan cheese

1. Preheat oven to 450°.
2. Combine potatoes and oil; toss to coat. Arrange potatoes, cut sides down, in a single layer on a parchment paper–lined baking sheet. Bake at 450° for 20 minutes. Turn potatoes; bake 10 minutes. Remove and cool 20 minutes.
3. Preheat broiler.
4. Using a paring knife, carefully cut a circle in cut side of potatoes. Using a melon baller or small spoon, remove pulp from potato, leaving a thin shell. Combine pulp, sour cream, 1 tablespoon chives, and next 5 ingredients (through pepper). Fill potato shells with filling; sprinkle with cheese and 1 tablespoon chives.
5. Broil potatoes 2 minutes or until cheese is lightly browned.

YIELD | SERVES 12 (SERVING SIZE: 2 POTATO HALVES)

CALORIES 85; FAT 3.9g (sat 2.2g, mono 1.2g, poly 0.2g); PROTEIN 2g; CARB 10g; FIBER 1g; CHOL 6mg; IRON 0mg; SODIUM 182mg; CALC 20mg

Pan-Seared Mojo Potatoes

4	teaspoons olive oil, divided
1	pound fingerling potatoes, halved lengthwise
⅜	teaspoon salt
⅔	cup tightly packed cilantro
2	teaspoons lime juice
1	teaspoon white wine vinegar
¼	teaspoon black pepper
1	large garlic clove, chopped
¼	cup reduced-fat sour cream

1. Heat a skillet over medium-high heat. Add 1 tablespoon oil and potatoes; cook 6 minutes. Cover, reduce heat to medium, and cook 6 minutes.
2. Sprinkle potatoes with salt. Combine 1 teaspoon oil, cilantro, and next 4 ingredients (through garlic) in a blender. Blend until smooth. Stir into potatoes. Top with sour cream.

YIELD | SERVES 4

CALORIES 151; FAT 6.5g (sat 1.8g, mono 3.3g, poly 0.5g); PROTEIN 4g; CARB 20g; FIBER 2g; CHOL 8mg; IRON 1mg; SODIUM 280mg; CALC 44mg

Goat Cheese and Basil Polenta

3	cups water
1	cup dry polenta
3	ounces goat cheese (about ⅓ cup)
1	tablespoon chopped fresh basil
¼	teaspoon freshly ground black pepper
¼	teaspoon kosher salt

1. Bring 3 cups water to a boil in a medium saucepan. Gradually add polenta, stirring constantly with a whisk. Reduce heat to low; cook 7 minutes, stirring occasionally. Remove from heat; stir in goat cheese, basil, pepper, and salt.

YIELD | SERVES 4 (SERVING SIZE: ¾ CUP)

CALORIES 204; FAT 4.5g (sat 3.1g, mono 1g, poly 0.1g); PROTEIN 7g; CARB 32g; FIBER 1g; CHOL 10mg; IRON 2mg; SODIUM 198mg; CALC 32mg

Rustic Garlic Mashed Potatoes

2	pounds unpeeled baking potatoes, quartered lengthwise
1	garlic head, peeled
¾	cup hot 1% low-fat milk or dairy-free alternative
1½	tablespoons butter, melted
½	teaspoon salt
¼	teaspoon freshly ground black pepper

1. Place potatoes and garlic head in a saucepan filled with water to cover; bring to a boil. Reduce heat, and simmer 15 minutes or until potatoes are tender. Drain and transfer to a bowl; mash with hot milk, butter, salt, and pepper.

YIELD | SERVES 4 (SERVING SIZE: ABOUT 1 CUP)

CALORIES 259; FAT 5g (sat 3.1g, mono 1.3g, poly 0.3g); PROTEIN 7g; CARB 48g; FIBER 3g; CHOL 14mg; IRON 2mg; SODIUM 363mg; CALC 116mg

Garlic-Parmesan Rice

- 1 tablespoon olive oil
- 1 garlic clove, minced
- 1 cup uncooked basmati rice
- 2 cups water
- 1 tablespoon chopped fresh flat-leaf parsley
- ¼ teaspoon kosher salt
- ⅛ teaspoon black pepper
- 1 ounce grated fresh Parmesan cheese (about ¼ cup)

1. Heat a saucepan over medium heat. Add oil to pan. Add garlic; sauté 30 seconds. Add rice; cook 1 minute, stirring constantly. Add 2 cups water; bring to a boil. Cover, reduce heat, and simmer 12 minutes or until liquid is absorbed. Remove from heat. Let stand 5 minutes. Stir in parsley, salt, pepper, and cheese.

YIELD | SERVES 4 (SERVING SIZE: ABOUT ¾ CUP)

CALORIES 242; FAT 5.4g (sat 1.7g, mono 3.1g, poly 0.4g); PROTEIN 5g; CARB 46g; FIBER 1g; CHOL 6mg; IRON 2mg; SODIUM 229mg; CALC 82mg

Wild Rice with Squash

- 5 cups water
- ⅔ cup uncooked wild rice
- 1½ tablespoons olive oil
- 1½ cups (½-inch) cubed peeled butternut squash
- 1 teaspoon chopped fresh rosemary
- ⅜ teaspoon salt, divided
- 1 shallot, chopped
- ⅛ teaspoon freshly ground black pepper

1. Place 5 cups water and rice in a saucepan; bring to a boil. Cover, reduce heat, and simmer 30 minutes. Turn off heat; let stand, covered, 25 minutes. Drain. Heat a skillet over medium heat; add oil. Add squash, rosemary, ⅛ teaspoon salt, and shallot; cook 10 minutes. Add rice, pepper, and ¼ teaspoon salt to squash mixture, stirring to combine.

YIELD | SERVES 4 (SERVING SIZE: ABOUT 1 CUP)

CALORIES 169; FAT 5.4g (sat 0.8g, mono 3.7g, poly 0.7g); PROTEIN 5g; CARB 27g; FIBER 3g; CHOL 0mg; IRON 1mg; SODIUM 185mg; CALC 34mg

Yogurt Rice with Cumin and Chile

Using whole packages of rice and yogurt saves the time of measuring. Be sure to use standard yogurt here; Greek is a bit too thick. Serve with grilled lamb chops, roasted chicken, or grilled salmon.

2	(8.5-ounce) pouches precooked white basmati rice (such as Uncle Ben's)
1	tablespoon canola oil
1	tablespoon bottled minced fresh ginger
1	teaspoon cumin seeds
1	serrano chile, thinly sliced
2	tablespoons chopped fresh cilantro
¾	teaspoon kosher salt
1	(6-ounce) carton plain low-fat yogurt

1. Heat rice according to package directions.

2. Heat a large skillet over medium-high heat. Add oil; swirl to coat. Add ginger, cumin, and chile; sauté 30 seconds. Stir in rice, cilantro, salt, and yogurt; cook 1 minute.

YIELD | SERVES 6 (SERVING SIZE: ½ CUP)

CALORIES 173; FAT 4.6g (sat 0.8g, mono 2.1g, poly 1.4g); PROTEIN 5g; CARB 29g; FIBER 1g; CHOL 2mg; IRON 1mg; SODIUM 265mg; CALC 56mg

DESSERT IS AN IMPORTANT PART OF ANY DIET, INCLUDING THIS ONE.

While something sweet doesn't need to be part of every meal, satisfying your cravings will actually help keep you on track with your weight loss. These recipes offer healthier options that don't have the excess calories and saturated fat that many ready-made gluten-free desserts do. Just remember that moderation is key.

Pineapple Upside-Down Cake

½   **cup packed brown sugar**
¼   **cup unsalted butter, divided**
1   **vanilla bean, split lengthwise**
6   **(½-inch-thick) slices fresh pineapple**
¼   **cup dark rum**
Cooking spray
5   **ounces gluten-free all-purpose flour (about 1 cup)**
0.9   **ounces almond meal flour (about ¼ cup)**
½   **teaspoon baking powder**
½   **teaspoon kosher salt**
¼   **teaspoon baking soda**
½   **cup light sour cream**
2   **tablespoons canola oil**
⅔   **cup granulated sugar**
2   **large eggs**

1. Preheat oven to 350°.

2. Combine brown sugar, 2 tablespoons butter, and vanilla bean in a skillet over medium heat; cook 6 minutes or until butter melts and sugar dissolves, stirring frequently. Add pineapple in a single layer. Carefully pour rum over pineapple; tilt pan to ignite. Simmer 5 minutes on each side or until slightly tender and caramelized. Remove vanilla bean.

3. Coat a 9-inch round cake pan with cooking spray. Arrange pineapple in a single layer in bottom of pan; pour sugar mixture over pineapple, tilting pan to coat bottom.

4. Weigh or lightly spoon flours into dry measuring cups; level with a knife. Combine flours, baking powder, salt, and baking soda. Melt 2 tablespoons butter in a microwave-safe dish at HIGH 35 seconds. Combine melted butter, sour cream, and oil in a bowl.

5. Beat granulated sugar and eggs with a mixer at high speed 5 minutes or until fluffy. Reduce speed to medium. Add flour mixture and sour cream mixture alternately to egg mixture, beginning and ending with flour mixture. Spread batter over pineapple. Bake at 350° for 38 minutes or until a wooden pick inserted in center comes out clean. Cool in pan 15 minutes on a wire rack.

YIELD | SERVES 10 (SERVING SIZE: 1 WEDGE)

CALORIES 292; FAT 11.2g (sat 4.4g, mono 3.7g, poly 1.2g); PROTEIN 4g; CARB 44g; FIBER 1g; CHOL 54mg; IRON 1mg; SODIUM 177mg; CALC 87mg

INGREDIENT TIP

Cooking with alcohol

The rum will ignite when you tilt the pan; this burns off most of the alcohol but leaves a delicious flavor behind.

Cocoa Cupcakes

2.1 ounces sweet white sorghum flour (about ½ cup)
1.15 ounces brown rice flour (about ¼ cup)
1.05 ounces tapioca flour (about ¼ cup)
½ cup unsweetened cocoa
1 teaspoon xanthan gum
½ teaspoon baking soda
½ teaspoon baking powder
½ teaspoon salt
¾ cup granulated sugar
¼ cup unsalted butter, softened
2 large eggs
1 cup fat-free sour cream
½ teaspoon vanilla extract
Cooking spray
1 cup powdered sugar
2 tablespoons unsalted butter, softened
1 tablespoon 1% low-fat milk
½ teaspoon vanilla extract

1. Preheat oven to 375°.
2. Weigh or lightly spoon flours into dry measuring cups; level with a knife. Combine flours, cocoa, and next 4 ingredients (through salt) in a medium bowl; stir with a whisk.
3. Place granulated sugar and ¼ cup butter in a large bowl; beat with a mixer at medium speed until blended. Add eggs, 1 at a time, beating well after each addition. Beat in sour cream and ½ teaspoon vanilla. Gradually add flour mixture, beating at low speed until smooth (batter will be very thick).
4. Place 12 paper muffin cup liners in muffin cups; coat liners with cooking spray. Spoon batter into prepared cups (cups will be almost full). Bake at 375° for 20 minutes or until a wooden pick inserted in center comes out clean. Cool in pan 10 minutes on a wire rack; remove from pan. Cool completely on wire rack.
5. Combine powdered sugar, 2 tablespoons butter, milk, and ½ teaspoon vanilla in a medium bowl; beat with a mixer at low speed until blended. Increase speed to medium; beat until smooth. Spread frosting over cupcakes.

YIELD | SERVES 12 (SERVING SIZE: 1 CUPCAKE)

CALORIES 218; FAT 7.7g (sat 4.4g, mono 2.1g, poly 0.4g); PROTEIN 4g; CARB 36g; FIBER 2g; CHOL 48mg; IRON 1mg; SODIUM 199mg; CALC 57mg

Blackberry-Almond Cobbler

4 cups fresh blackberries
3 tablespoons sugar
1 tablespoon cornstarch
1 tablespoon fresh lemon juice
Cooking spray
2.3 ounces brown rice flour (about ½ cup)
1.8 ounces almond meal flour (about ½ cup)
¼ cup sugar
1 teaspoon baking powder
⅛ teaspoon salt
1 large egg, beaten
4 tablespoons butter, melted and cooled
2 cups vanilla light ice cream

1. Preheat oven to 375°.

2. Place blackberries in a large bowl; add 3 tablespoons sugar, cornstarch, and juice, stirring to coat berries. Pour mixture into an 8-inch square glass or ceramic baking dish coated with cooking spray.

3. Weigh or lightly spoon flours into dry measuring cups; level with a knife. Combine flours, ¼ cup sugar, baking powder, and salt in a large bowl, stirring with a whisk. Add egg, stirring to combine. Add butter, stirring just until moist.

4. Drop batter by teaspoonfuls onto blackberry mixture. Bake at 375° for 30 minutes or until topping is lightly browned. Cool 10 minutes. Serve with ice cream.

YIELD | SERVES 8 (SERVING SIZE: ⅛ OF COBBLER AND ¼ CUP ICE CREAM)

CALORIES 276; FAT 12.2g (sat 5.3g, mono 2.5g, poly 0.7g); PROTEIN 6g; CARB 38g; FIBER 5g; CHOL 49mg; IRON 1mg; SODIUM 183mg; CALC 143mg

Grilled Peaches with Honey Cream

You can use apricots or nectarines instead of peaches.

- 2 tablespoons unsalted butter, melted
- 2 tablespoons honey, divided
- ¼ teaspoon ground cardamom
- Dash of kosher salt
- 4 medium peaches, pitted and halved
- Cooking spray
- ⅓ cup plain fat-free Greek yogurt
- 2½ tablespoons half-and-half
- ¼ teaspoon vanilla extract
- 1 cup raspberries
- Mint leaves (optional)

1. Combine butter, 1 tablespoon honey, cardamom, and salt in a medium bowl. Add peaches, and toss to coat. Let stand 5 minutes.

2. Heat a grill pan over medium heat. Coat pan with cooking spray. Arrange peaches on grill pan; grill 2 minutes on each side or until grill marks appear.

3. Combine yogurt, half-and-half, 1 tablespoon honey, and vanilla in a small bowl; stir with a whisk. Serve with peaches and raspberries. Garnish with mint leaves, if desired.

YIELD | SERVES 4 (SERVING SIZE: 2 PEACH HALVES, ¼ CUP RASPBERRIES, AND 2 TABLESPOONS YOGURT MIXTURE)

CALORIES 182; FAT 7.6g (sat 4.4g, mono 1.6g, poly 0.5g); PROTEIN 4g; CARB 28g; FIBER 4g; CHOL 19mg; IRON 1mg; SODIUM 43mg; CALC 42mg

Meyer Lemon Panna Cotta

Meyer lemon—a lemon/orange hybrid—is sweeter than conventional lemon. If you don't have access to Meyer lemons, you can use a regular lemon and enjoy a dessert that's a bit more tart.

- 1 Meyer or regular lemon
- ½ cup plus 3 tablespoons 2% reduced-fat milk, divided
- ½ cup half-and-half
- ⅓ cup sugar
- ¼ teaspoon salt
- 1¾ teaspoons unflavored gelatin
- 1½ cups low-fat buttermilk
- Cooking spray
- Mint leaves and lemon rind strips (optional)

1. Remove rind from lemon using a vegetable peeler, avoiding white pith. Squeeze 3 tablespoons juice from lemon. Combine rind, ½ cup reduced-fat milk, half-and-half, sugar, and salt in a small saucepan; bring to a simmer over medium heat (do not boil). Remove pan from heat; cover and let stand 20 minutes. Discard rind. Sprinkle gelatin over 3 tablespoons reduced-fat milk in a small bowl, and let stand at least 10 minutes.

2. Return half-and-half mixture to medium heat; cook 1 minute or until very hot. Add gelatin mixture, stirring with a whisk until dissolved (about 1 minute). Stir in buttermilk and 3 tablespoons juice. Divide mixture among 4 (6-ounce) ramekins or custard cups coated with cooking spray. Cover and refrigerate 4 hours.

3. Run a knife around outside edges of each panna cotta. Place a plate upside down on top of each cup; invert panna cotta onto plate. Garnish with mint and lemon rind strips, if desired.

YIELD | SERVES 4

CALORIES 185; FAT 6.3g (sat 3.8g, mono 0.8g, poly 0.1g); PROTEIN 7g; CARB 26g; FIBER 0g; CHOL 22mg; IRON 0mg; SODIUM 258mg; CALC 214mg

Chocolate–Peanut Butter Pudding

⅓	cup sugar	2	ounces milk chocolate, finely chopped
2	tablespoons cornstarch	¼	cup creamy peanut butter
2	tablespoons Dutch process cocoa	1	tablespoon chopped unsalted, dry-roasted peanuts
1½	cups 1% low-fat milk		
½	cup light cream		

1. Combine sugar, cornstarch, and cocoa in a medium saucepan; stir with a whisk. Whisk in milk and cream. Bring to a boil over medium-high heat. Cook 1 minute or until thick and bubbly. Remove from heat. Add chocolate and peanut butter, stirring until smooth. Spoon about ⅓ cup pudding into each of 6 bowls. Top each serving with ½ teaspoon peanuts.

YIELD | SERVES 6

CALORIES 245; FAT 13.7g (sat 5.4g, mono 3.8g, poly 1.9g); PROTEIN 6g; CARB 27g; FIBER 1g; CHOL 12mg; IRON 1mg; SODIUM 104mg; CALC 123mg

Butterscotch Pudding

½	cup packed dark brown sugar	1	tablespoon butter
3½	tablespoons cornstarch	2	teaspoons vanilla extract
⅛	teaspoon salt		Cooking spray
2	cups 1% low-fat milk	5	teaspoons almond brickle chips (such as Heath)
2	large egg yolks, lightly beaten		

1. Combine brown sugar, cornstarch, and salt in a medium saucepan over medium heat. Add milk and egg yolks, stirring with a whisk until smooth.
2. Bring mixture to a boil, and cook 2 to 3 minutes or until mixture thickens, stirring constantly.
3. Remove pan from heat; stir in butter and vanilla. Pour mixture into 5 (6-ounce) ramekins or small bowls. Cover surface of pudding with plastic wrap coated with cooking spray; cool 15 minutes. Chill at least 4 hours. Top each serving with 1 teaspoon brickle chips.

YIELD | SERVES 5

CALORIES 220; FAT 6.6g (sat 3.4g, mono 1.7g, poly 0.4g); PROTEIN 5g; CARB 35g; FIBER 0g; CHOL 86mg; IRON 0mg; SODIUM 152mg; CALC 150mg

Jasmine Chai Rice Pudding

Although it keeps several days in the fridge, this pudding is at its best warm. Add a touch of extra milk to reheat, and top with whipped topping, nuts, and rind just before serving.

2	cups 1% low-fat milk, divided
1½	cups water
2	teaspoons loose chai tea (about 4 tea bags)
⅛	teaspoon salt
1	cup uncooked jasmine rice
¾	cup sweetened condensed milk
¼	cup diced dried mixed fruit
2	large egg yolks
1	tablespoon butter
6	tablespoons frozen fat-free whipped topping, thawed
2	tablespoons chopped pistachios
½	teaspoon grated orange rind

1. Combine 1 cup low-fat milk, 1½ cups water, tea, and salt in a large saucepan; bring to a boil. Remove from heat; steep 1 minute. Strain milk mixture through a fine sieve into a bowl; discard solids. Return milk mixture to pan; place pan over medium heat. Stir in rice. Cover and simmer 10 minutes. Combine 1 cup low-fat milk, condensed milk, fruit, and egg yolks, stirring well with a whisk. Gradually add half of hot milk mixture to egg yolk mixture, stirring constantly with a whisk. Return milk mixture to pan; cook 10 minutes or until mixture is thick and rice is tender, stirring constantly. Remove from heat; stir in butter.

2. Place ⅔ cup rice pudding in each of 6 bowls. Top each serving with 1 tablespoon whipped topping. Combine nuts and rind. Sprinkle about 1 teaspoon nut mixture over each serving.

YIELD | SERVES 6

CALORIES 287; FAT 8.8g (sat 4.5g, mono 3g, poly 0.8g); PROTEIN 8g; CARB 44g; FIBER 1g; CHOL 90mg; IRON 1mg; SODIUM 169mg; CALC 223mg

Almond-Date Bars

Marcona almonds are blanched and roasted—you won't need to toast them. You can also substitute regular whole almonds. For the best texture, use whole pitted dates, not chopped; you need the sticky texture of the whole fruit.

- 1¼ cups pitted dates (about 15)
- 1 cup Marcona almonds
- ¾ cup dried apples (about 2 ounces)
- ¼ cup flaked sweetened coconut
- 1 tablespoon honey
- ⅛ teaspoon kosher salt
- ¾ cup crispy rice cereal
- Cooking spray

1. Place first 6 ingredients in the bowl of a food processor; process until finely chopped. Add cereal; pulse to combine. Press date mixture into bottom of an 8-inch square glass or ceramic baking dish coated with cooking spray. Cut into 12 pieces.

YIELD | SERVES 12 (SERVING SIZE: 1 BAR)

CALORIES 142; FAT 6.3g (sat 1g, mono 3.7g, poly 1.5g); PROTEIN 3g; CARB 22g; FIBER 3g; CHOL 0mg; IRON 1mg; SODIUM 76mg; CALC 36mg

Maple-Pecan Bars

- 2.6 ounces white rice flour (about ½ cup)
- 2.3 ounces cornstarch (about ½ cup)
- 2.1 ounces sweet sorghum flour (about ½ cup)
- ½ cup packed brown sugar
- 6 tablespoons butter
- 1 teaspoon xanthan gum
- 2 teaspoons vanilla extract
- ¼ teaspoon salt
- ½ cup maple syrup
- ⅓ cup packed brown sugar
- ¼ cup 1% low-fat milk
- 1 tablespoon butter
- ½ cup whole pecans
- ½ teaspoon vanilla extract

1. Preheat oven to 375°. Line a 9-inch square metal baking pan with parchment paper.

2. Weigh or lightly spoon white rice flour, cornstarch, and sweet sorghum flour into dry measuring cups; level with a knife. Place white rice flour, cornstarch, sweet sorghum flour, ½ cup brown sugar, 6 tablespoons butter, xanthan gum, 2 teaspoons vanilla, and salt in a food processor; pulse until mixture resembles fine meal. Press flour mixture into bottom of prepared pan. Bake at 375° for 15 minutes or until edges of crust are lightly browned.

3. While crust bakes, combine syrup, ⅓ cup brown sugar, milk, and 1 tablespoon butter in a medium saucepan; bring to a boil over medium heat. Cook 2 minutes, stirring constantly with a whisk until sugar dissolves. Remove from heat; add pecans and ½ teaspoon vanilla, stirring with a whisk. Pour mixture into hot crust. Bake at 375° for 10 minutes or until filling is bubbly. Cool completely in pan. Cut into 20 bars.

YIELD | SERVES 20 (SERVING SIZE: 1 BAR)

CALORIES 149; **FAT** 6.2g (sat 2.8g, mono 2.2g, poly 0.8g); **PROTEIN** 1g; **CARB** 23g; **FIBER** 1g; **CHOL** 11mg; **IRON** 0mg; **SODIUM** 70mg; **CALC** 23mg

Lemon Sugar Cookies

The stark contrast between the sweet sugars and the tart lemon rind gives these cookies personality and bite. They're a great afternoon treat with coffee or tea.

- 2.3 ounces brown rice flour (about ½ cup)
- 1.8 ounces almond meal flour (about ½ cup)
- 1.05 ounces tapioca flour (about ¼ cup)
- 1.3 ounces potato starch (about ¼ cup)
- 1 teaspoon xanthan gum
- 1 teaspoon baking powder
- ¼ teaspoon salt
- 4 tablespoons butter, softened
- ½ cup granulated sugar
- ½ cup packed brown sugar
- 1 tablespoon fresh lemon juice
- 1 teaspoon vanilla extract
- ½ teaspoon grated lemon rind
- 2 large egg yolks

1. Preheat oven to 350°.

2. Weigh or lightly spoon flours and starch into dry measuring cups; level with a knife. Combine flours, potato starch, xanthan gum, baking powder, and salt in a medium bowl, stirring with a whisk.

3. Place butter and sugars in a bowl; beat with a mixer at medium speed until well blended. Add juice, vanilla, rind, and egg yolks; beat until blended. Add flour mixture, ¼ cup at a time, beating after each addition.

4. Cover a large baking sheet with parchment paper. Shape dough into 20 balls. Place 2 inches apart on baking sheet. Bake at 350° for 15 to 20 minutes or until lightly browned. Cool on pan 5 minutes. Remove cookies from pan; cool completely on wire racks.

YIELD | SERVES 20 (SERVING SIZE: 1 COOKIE)

CALORIES 105; FAT 4.1g (sat 1.7g, mono 0.8g, poly 0.2g); PROTEIN 1g; CARB 17g; FIBER 1g; CHOL 25mg; IRON 0mg; SODIUM 75mg; CALC 30mg

Peanut Butter–Chocolate Chip Cookies

You probably have everything on hand to make these chewy, chocolaty peanut butter cookies. To fit the cookies on a single sheet pan, divide cookies into five rows of four. Pressing the cookies flat helps them bake quickly and get lovely crisp edges; otherwise they'll be too round and undercooked.

- ¼ teaspoon salt
- 1 large egg white
- 1 cup reduced-fat chunky peanut butter
- ⅓ cup granulated sugar
- ¼ cup packed brown sugar
- ¼ cup semisweet chocolate minichips

1. Preheat oven to 375°.

2. Place salt and egg white in a medium bowl; stir with a whisk until white is frothy. Add peanut butter, granulated sugar, brown sugar, and chocolate chips, stirring to combine.

3. Divide dough into 20 equal portions (about 1 tablespoon each); arrange dough 2 inches apart on a baking sheet lined with parchment paper. Gently press the top of each cookie with a fork; press the top of each cookie again to form a crisscross pattern, and flatten to a 2-inch diameter. Bake at 375° for 10 minutes or until lightly browned.

YIELD | SERVES 20 (SERVING SIZE: 1 COOKIE)

CALORIES 111; FAT 5.6g (sat 1.4g, mono 2.6g, poly 1.4g); PROTEIN 3g; CARB 13g; FIBER 1g; CHOL 0mg; IRON 0mg; SODIUM 121mg; CALC 3mg

Amaretti

1 cup granulated sugar
1 (7-ounce) package almond paste
1 teaspoon amaretto (almond-flavored liqueur)

2 large egg whites
¼ cup turbinado sugar

1. Preheat oven to 350°.
2. Place granulated sugar and almond paste in a large bowl; beat with a mixer at medium speed until almond paste is broken into small pieces. Add amaretto and egg whites; beat at high speed 4 minutes or until smooth. Chill batter 20 minutes.
3. Drop batter by teaspoonfuls 1 inch apart on parchment paper–lined baking sheets. Sprinkle with turbinado sugar. Bake at 350° for 10 minutes or until edges of cookies are golden brown. Cool completely on pans; carefully remove cookies from parchment. Cool on wire racks.

YIELD | SERVES 40 (SERVING SIZE: 1 COOKIE)

CALORIES 48; FAT 1.4g (sat 0.1g, mono 0.9g, poly 0.3g); PROTEIN 1g; CARB 9g; FIBER 0g; CHOL 0mg; IRON 0mg; SODIUM 3mg; CALC 9mg

Lemon Verbena–Buttermilk Sherbet

1 cup granulated sugar
¾ cup water
3 tablespoons packed, coarsely chopped lemon verbena

2½ cups cold whole-milk buttermilk
1 tablespoon grated lemon rind
Dash of salt
Lemon rind strips (optional)

1. Combine first 3 ingredients in a saucepan, stirring until sugar dissolves. Bring to a boil; boil 2 minutes. Remove from heat; let stand 30 minutes. Pour syrup through a fine sieve into a bowl; discard solids. Stir in buttermilk, rind, and salt; chill 1 hour.
2. Pour mixture into the freezer can of an ice-cream freezer; freeze according to manufacturer's instructions. Spoon sherbet into a freezer-safe container; cover and freeze 1 hour or until firm. Garnish with lemon rind strips, if desired.

YIELD | SERVES 8 (SERVING SIZE: ABOUT ½ CUP)

CALORIES 145; FAT 2.5g (sat 1.5g, mono 0.6g, poly 0.2g); PROTEIN 2g; CARB 29g; FIBER 0g; CHOL 8mg; IRON 0mg; SODIUM 99mg; CALC 89mg

Cherry-Grapefruit-Basil Sorbet

1	cup water	3	cups pitted cherries
½	cup sugar	½	cup fresh ruby red grapefruit juice (about 1 grapefruit)
	Dash of kosher salt		
½	cup basil leaves	1½	teaspoons fresh lime juice

1. Combine first 3 ingredients in a small saucepan; bring to a boil, stirring until sugar dissolves. Stir in basil; remove from heat. Cover and let stand 30 minutes.

2. Place cherries in a food processor; process until smooth. Add syrup, grapefruit juice, and lime juice; process until well blended. Strain cherry mixture through a fine sieve over a bowl; discard solids. Pour cherry mixture into the freezer can of an ice-cream freezer; freeze according to manufacturer's instructions. Spoon sorbet into a freezer-safe container; cover and freeze 1 hour or until firm.

YIELD | SERVES 7 (SERVING SIZE: ½ CUP)

CALORIES 105; FAT 0.2g (sat 0g, mono 0g, poly 0.1g); PROTEIN 1g; CARB 27g; FIBER 1g; CHOL 0mg; IRON 0mg; SODIUM 18mg; CALC 16mg

Quick Berry Frozen Yogurt

2	cups frozen mixed berries, divided	¼	cup fat-free milk
1	cup vanilla low-fat frozen yogurt, divided	1	tablespoon chopped fresh mint
		1	tablespoon honey

1. Combine 1 cup berries, ¾ cup yogurt, milk, mint, and honey in the bowl of a food processor; process until smooth. Spoon into a freezer-safe container. Add 1 cup berries and ¼ cup yogurt to processor; process until smooth. Swirl berry mixture into yogurt mixture. Serve immediately, or freeze until firm.

YIELD | SERVES 4 (SERVING SIZE: ABOUT ½ CUP)

CALORIES 150; FAT 2.5g (sat 1.3g, mono 0.4g, poly 0.2g); PROTEIN 6g; CARB 29g; FIBER 2g; CHOL 33mg; IRON 0mg; SODIUM 34mg; CALC 155mg

Blueberry Cheesecake Ice Cream

2 cups granulated sugar
6 ounces ⅓-less-fat cream cheese, softened (about ¾ cup)
4 large egg yolks
3 cups 2% reduced-fat milk
1 cup half-and-half
3 cups fresh blueberries, coarsely chopped
¼ cup powdered sugar
¼ cup water

1. Combine first 3 ingredients in a large bowl; beat with a mixer at high speed until smooth. Combine milk and half-and-half in a medium, heavy saucepan; bring to a boil. Remove from heat. Gradually add half of hot milk mixture to cheese mixture, stirring constantly with a whisk. Return milk mixture to pan. Cook over medium-low heat 5 minutes or until a thermometer registers 160°, stirring constantly. Place pan in an ice-filled bowl. Cool completely, stirring occasionally.
2. Combine blueberries, powdered sugar, and ¼ cup water in a small saucepan; bring to a boil. Reduce heat, and simmer 10 minutes or until mixture thickens slightly, stirring frequently. Remove from heat, and cool completely.
3. Stir blueberry mixture into milk mixture. Pour mixture into the freezer can of an ice-cream freezer; freeze according to manufacturer's instructions. Spoon ice cream into a freezer-safe container; cover and freeze 1 hour or until firm.

Note: This recipe yields 2 quarts of ice cream, so if you make the entire recipe, use a traditional bucket-style freezer. Halve the recipe if you use a countertop model; they typically have a smaller capacity.

YIELD | SERVES 12 (SERVING SIZE: ABOUT ⅔ CUP)

CALORIES 268; FAT 7.8g (sat 4.4g, mono 2.3g, poly 0.5g); PROTEIN 5g; CARB 46g; FIBER 1g; CHOL 90mg; IRON 0mg; SODIUM 100mg; CALC 49mg

Raspberries with Peach-Basil Sorbet

Here's a twist on peach Melba, the classic dessert of poached peaches with raspberry sauce. We turn juicy summer peaches instead into a velvety sorbet spiked with basil and serve it with fresh raspberries for the perfect ending to a summer meal.

1 cup granulated sugar
¾ cup water
¼ cup packed, coarsely chopped fresh basil leaves
1½ pounds ripe peaches
1 tablespoon fresh lemon juice
Dash of salt
12 ounces fresh raspberries
Basil sprigs (optional)

1. Combine first 3 ingredients in a saucepan. Bring to a boil; stir until sugar dissolves. Let stand 15 minutes. Pour through a fine sieve into a bowl; discard solids.

2. Cook peaches in a large pot of boiling water 1 minute. Place peaches in a bowl of ice water until cool. Peel peaches; remove pits and chop flesh. Place chopped peaches and juice in a blender; process until smooth. Stir peach mixture and salt into basil mixture. Chill 1 hour.

3. Pour peach mixture into the freezer can of an ice-cream freezer; freeze according to manufacturer's instructions. Spoon sorbet into a freezer-safe container; cover and freeze until firm. Serve with raspberries. Garnish with basil sprigs, if desired.

YIELD | SERVES 6 (SERVING SIZE: ½ CUP SORBET AND ABOUT ⅓ CUP RASPBERRIES)

CALORIES 199; FAT 0.6g (sat 0g, mono 0.1g, poly 0.3g); PROTEIN 2g; CARB 50g; FIBER 5g; CHOL 0mg; IRON 1mg; SODIUM 26mg; CALC 21mg

Watermelon with Tangy Granita

1 cup water	¼ teaspoon crushed red pepper
¾ cup sugar	1 tablespoon grated lime rind
½ cup fresh lime juice	1 cucumber, peeled and seeded
⅓ cup packed mint leaves	8 cups (¾-inch) cubed watermelon
⅓ cup packed cilantro leaves	½ teaspoon kosher salt
¼ teaspoon kosher salt	

1. Combine 1 cup water and sugar in a microwave-safe dish. Microwave at HIGH 2 minutes; cool completely. Place syrup, juice, and next 6 ingredients (through cucumber) in a blender; blend until smooth. Pour mixture into an 11 x 7–inch glass or ceramic baking dish; cover and freeze 3 hours or until firm, stirring with a fork every 45 minutes. Remove mixture from freezer; scrape entire mixture with a fork until fluffy.

2. Place watermelon cubes in a large bowl. Sprinkle with salt; toss to combine. Let stand 10 minutes. Spoon about 1½ cups watermelon mixture into each of 6 bowls; top each serving with about ½ cup granita.

YIELD | SERVES 6

CALORIES 170; FAT 0.4g (sat 0g, mono 0.1g, poly 0.1g); PROTEIN 2g; CARB 43g; FIBER 1g; CHOL 0mg; IRON 0mg; SODIUM 244mg; CALC 25mg

Cantaloupe Granita

4 cups cubed peeled cantaloupe	2 tablespoons fresh lime juice
⅓ cup agave nectar	⅛ teaspoon salt

1. Place cantaloupe in a food processor or blender; process until smooth. Strain through a fine sieve over a bowl; discard solids. Stir in nectar, juice, and salt. Pour mixture into an 8-inch square glass or ceramic baking dish. Freeze at least 8 hours. Remove mixture from freezer; scrape entire mixture with a fork until fluffy.

YIELD | SERVES 4 (SERVING SIZE: ABOUT 1 CUP)

CALORIES 136; FAT 0.3g (sat 0.1g, mono 0g, poly 0.1g); PROTEIN 1g; CARB 35g; FIBER 1g; CHOL 0mg; IRON 0mg; SODIUM 100mg; CALC 15mg

PART 3

LIVING THE GLUTEN-FREE LIFESTYLE

EXERCISING FOR GLUTEN-FREE HEALTH

F YOU REALLY WANT TO BENEFIT from your gluten-free diet, exercise is a necessary step. As you shift your diet to this approach, your body will crave and respond to a routine that helps you get—and stay—fit. You'll be happy to learn that you won't have to trudge on a treadmill for hours or start scheduling marathons. In fact, if you're a regular exerciser you'll discover in these pages that you can probably exercise for less time *and* get better results.

Pairing your pure-energy eating plan with this fitness approach will do wonders for your body and your weight loss. The first step is to start building more activity into your typical day. For example, if you work in an office, try out a standing desk. Or, if that's not possible, look for opportunities to stand and move whenever possible. This could mean taking all your calls while standing or answering interoffice messages in person. Instead of tapping out an email or instant message, get up and walk over to your correspondent. You'll not only get more activity, but your officemates will probably appreciate the face-to-face contact.

As for actual exercise, make it your goal to find active ways to play so that your workouts never feel like an obligation. The problem with our modern-day exercise is that it's usually one more chore out of many, and we happily put it off when something—anything—better presents itself. For that reason, you'll want to find activities that you love so much that you can't bear *not* doing them.

The reason playing games—or just playing—works so well is that it usually involves quick bursts and brief rests. Think about most of the physical games we play: Tennis, racquetball, basketball, soccer—they all require quick explosive efforts broken up by brief rests. The great thing about this approach to exercise is that you can include tag and wrestling with the kids or a pet. The ideal exercise involves brief intense bursts, like running after a ball or pursuing someone, that are broken up with pauses in the action that allow you to catch your breath, such as when you're between points or rallies or while you're taking a break on the grass.

Why is this start-stop approach important? Researchers have found that breaking up your activity like this leads to more weight loss and improved fitness. Exercise scientists refer to this type of exercise as HIIT: high-intensity interval training. In study after study, researchers have found it far outperforms standard, steady-paced cardio. Another plus is that exercising this way is more fun.

In a 2011 study published in the *Journal of Obesity*, researchers reviewed all the research available on HIIT, or interval-based exercise, and found that it trumped steady-paced exercise in all the measures studied. Interval training increased fitness and fat loss more than regular exercise, and it accomplished these results in about half the time. (A typical interval-based workout runs 20 to 30 minutes, while steady-paced sessions usually run 40 to 60 minutes.) Even better for dieters, in one study, researchers found interval training led to at least three times the weight loss of steady-paced aerobics. Interval training also seems to target abdominal fat—your belly—which envelops organs and can lead to chronic disease.

There are more benefits to interval training. According to the American College of Sports Medicine, you can elevate your metabolism for up to 24 hours post-exercise by doing intervals. By injecting brief periods of intense effort into your exercise (either by playing fast-paced games or adding in some jogging and sprinting into your regular walks, runs, swims, or cycling), you can kick your metabolism up a notch during your workout—and it takes hours for it to slow down again. That equals ongoing calorie burn long after you've showered and toweled off.

Adding Intervals to Your Workout

Obviously, the best way to build in interval training is to pick up a sport that naturally requires brief bursts of intense effort. But you can't play tennis or basketball all the time. You may not even enjoy competitive sports.

Don't worry. You can still make intervals part of your workout by mixing them into your usual pursuit. If you're a walker and you typically exercise for 30 minutes, every five minutes try adding a burst of jogging or fast walking for 30 seconds. As you become more fit, you can increase the interval length to a minute and decrease the walking segments to four minutes. For the biggest metabolism boost, you'll want to make sure that the interval portion leaves you breathing hard. (By the way, if you haven't been exercising regularly, check with your doctor before you start an interval program.)

You can set a goal of working toward a more challenging interval sequence, at least according to science. Referred to as "10-20-30"—or more accurately, "30-20-10"—the concept is that after a proper warmup, you do 30 seconds of whatever your activity—walking, jogging, swimming, etc.—at a light, easy-to-maintain pace. Then do 20 seconds of normal-level intensity, and end the minute with 10 seconds of all-out effort before going back to 30 seconds of light effort. The advantage of this approach is that after five to 10 minutes, you'll get a very thorough and demanding workout. You can go longer, of course, but just 10 minutes of this leads to improved stamina and lower blood pressure and cholesterol, according to the Danish researchers at the University of Copenhagen who developed this approach.

Beef Up Your Exercise

The other important aspect of any exercise program is building strength. All activity prescriptions from fitness experts include strength training. Again, there's news here that will help you shorten the length of time you spend lifting while providing you with better results. This program will shape and tone your body while helping you shed more pounds—and keep them off.

Instead of doing three sets of light lifts and spending hours and days in the gym, think about doing briefer, more intense weight lifting. You don't even need equipment; you could use the resistance provided by your own body weight to create a complete full-body regimen. Push-ups, pull-ups, crunches, lunges, squats, and calf raises, and you're done.

However, many people find that going to a gym can help them stay committed to a program. Check out Bodypump or cardio-strength classes to simulate the kind of strength regimen you're looking for, or explore more old-school techniques like using kettlebells or CrossFit.

Strength training definitely helps you shed pounds faster while making your body look better. In 2010, Australian researchers reported that when overweight dieters added strength training three times a week, they lost much more weight than people who only dieted. After four months, the strength-training group had dropped an average of 30 pounds—10 pounds more than dieters. What's more, the lifters shaved 5.5 inches off their waistlines, compared to just 3.5 inches in the diet-only group. The exercises included just eight moves: shoulder, chest, tricep, and leg presses; seated rows; knee extensions; lat pull-downs; and sit-ups. You can approximate most of these lifts (or variations of them) at home with a pair of dumbbells.

Pulling off a workout with these kinds of benefits may mean lifting heavier weights than most people typically do (or want to). How much weight is enough? In the program below, you'll do two sets of each move. You should choose a weight heavy enough so that your muscles are spent after the second set.

Complete two sets of eight to 12 repetitions with a one-minute rest between sets. Schedule workouts at least twice a week, but make sure you have a day off between sessions to give your muscles a chance to recover.

1. Chest press
2. Dumbbell lunge
3. Shoulder press
4. Crunches
5. Calf raises
6. Dumbbell squat
7. Biceps curl
8. Triceps kickback

Chest press

1. Lie on the floor faceup with your feet firmly on the ground, your back relaxed. Grasp a pair of dumbbells and with arms bent hold the dumbbells above your chest with your palms facing forward and your thumbs wrapped around each weight.

2. Exhale and slowly press the dumbbells straight up so they are over your shoulders. Wrists should remain in a neutral position (do not bend them throughout the exercise). Be careful not to arch your back. Inhale as you slowly lower the dumbbells back to starting position.

Dumbbell lunge

1. Stand with your feet hip-width apart, toes facing forward. Grasp a light dumbbell in each hand. Brace your torso by contracting your abdominal muscles. Slowly step forward with the right leg, placing your foot firmly on the ground. Keep your torso upright.

2. Inhale and bend your knees to lower your body toward the floor. Lunge only as far as you feel comfortable or until your right thigh is parallel to the floor. Now, exhale and firmly push off with your right (front) leg and return to your starting position. Repeat with the left leg.

Note: This exercise can also be done without weights.

Shoulder press

1. Hold a dumbbell in each hand, and stand with your feet hip-width apart. Brace your torso by contracting your abdominal muscles. Exhale and slowly lift the dumbbells until they are level with your shoulders. Palms should be facing in and thumbs should be wrapped around the handles. Wrists should remain in a neutral position (do not bend them throughout the exercise). Pull your shoulder blades down and back.

2. Exhale and press the dumbbells overhead until your elbows are straight, taking care not to arch your back. Inhale and slowly lower the dumbbells to shoulder height.

Crunches

1. Lie faceup on the floor with your knees bent, feet flat on the floor, and heels a comfortable distance away from your rear. Grasp a dumbbell vertically against your chest with both hands.

2. Engage your abdominal muscles and exhale as you slowly raise your head and shoulders off the floor and draw your rib cage toward your pelvis. Continue until your mid back is lifted off the floor. Pause at the top of the motion; then slowly lower your head and shoulders back to the mat as you inhale. Repeat for 60 seconds.

Note: This exercise can also be done without weights.

Calf raises

1. Stand holding a dumbbell in each hand. Spread your feet so they are hip-width apart. Keep your back straight and tighten your abs.

2. Exhale and slowly rise onto the balls of your feet, keeping your knees straight but not locked. At the top, pause and squeeze your calves. Inhale and lower yourself to the ground. Repeat step 2.

Note: This exercise can also be done without weights.

Dumbbell squat

1. Grasp a dumbbell vertically in front of your chest with both hands, and point elbows to the floor. Spread feet until they are hip-width apart.

2. Inhale and squat by slowly pushing back your hips and bending your knees. Squat only as low as you feel comfortable or until your thighs are parallel to the floor. Pause; then exhale and slowly return to starting position.

Note: This exercise can also be done without weights.

Biceps curl

1. Stand with your feet hip-width apart and grasp a pair of dumbbells with palms facing forward and your thumbs wrapped around each weight. Keep your back straight, your abdominals tight, and your shoulders down and back.

2. Bending at your elbows, exhale and pull the dumbbells directly up until they are level with the top of your chest. Pause at the top of the movement. Inhale and slowly lower the dumbbells to the starting position.

Triceps kickback

1. Grasp a pair of dumbbells with palms facing toward each other, thumbs wrapped around each weight. Spread your feet so they are hip-width apart and lean slightly forward, allowing dumbbells to hang.

2. Exhale and bend your right elbow and draw the dumbbell up to your side, making your upper arm parallel with the floor. Extend the dumbbell back to bring your forearm in line with your upper arm. Inhale and reverse the movement slowly by bending your elbow. Do 12 to 15 reps with each arm.

MAINTAIN YOUR GAINS THE GLUTEN-FREE WAY

ONE OF THE MOST **COMMON DOWNFALLS** of successful dieters is thinking that maintaining weight loss will draw on the same skills it took to lose the weight in the first place. Unfortunately, that's just not true. According to health statistics from the CDC, only 20 percent of the people who go on a diet manage to maintain their weight loss for more than a year.

The trouble is that the skills we rely on to lose weight aren't all that useful when it comes to maintaining our weight loss. A 2011 national survey from researchers at universities around the United States—Penn State, Drexel, Ohio State, Stanford, and Texas—has found several distinct strategies to losing weight, and they're different from the ones we need to keep the pounds off.

Published in the *American Journal of Preventive Medicine*, the study suggests it's not simply a lack of willpower or self-control. Christopher Sciamanna, M.D., the study's lead author, queried 1,165 people about the behaviors they relied on to lose weight and, among those who were successful losers (they had kept off at least 10 percent of their weight for a year or more), how they had maintained that loss. Sciamanna and his colleagues found that out of 36 specific practices used for short-term and long-term weight loss, 14 were specific to either the dieting phase or the maintenance phase, but not both. Yet these were the most valuable strategies, since they were most likely to predict success in either losing weight or keeping it off.

Nearly every study shows that weight loss peaks and regain starts at six months, points out Sciamanna, a professor of medicine and public health at Penn State College of Medicine. He's hopeful that the study findings can alter this pattern. While many of the key practices sound familiar, Sciamanna's research is the first to distinguish the role each plays in weight loss versus weight maintenance. Several of the strategies Sciamanna looked at worked for both the active weight-loss phase and maintenance. These are the behaviors you'll want to learn early and retain for the rest of your life:

- Eating plenty of lean sources of protein, like fish, lean beef, and poultry
- Eating plenty of fruits and vegetables
- Limiting carbohydrates, especially junky ones such as chips and donuts
- Keeping careful control of portions
- Following a regular exercise routine
- Writing out—and sticking to—your grocery list
- Paying attention to nutrition labels and avoiding processed foods
- Reminding and rewarding yourself for reaching and sustaining a healthy weight
- Weighing yourself regularly

Sciamanna's findings on weight-loss strategies can serve as something of a road map to long-term success. But it's important to realize that you have to continue to pursue behaviors that will help you stay trim. Sciamanna points out that obesity is a chronic illness like hypertension; no one is surprised when a hypertensive patient stops taking her medication and her blood pressure rises, so it should be no surprise that when you stop using weight-control practices the weight will come back all the same, he says. We'll explore these valuable techniques and how they relate to your plan.

Keep Eating Gluten Free?

Once the weight comes off, you may be wondering whether you can or should continue to follow a gluten-free plan. After all, you're omitting big food groups—do you need to abandon them for life?

You may not need to be quite as strict about your gluten-free diet down the road—it all depends on how well the diet is working for you and how much you miss some of the foods you've given up. The decision is entirely up to you. If you're really craving bread, try adding a serving or two a week to see how your body responds. Try it for breakfast on a Monday and pay close attention to what your body does: If you find that you feel bloated later that day, you might want to continue avoiding gluten.

If you decide to have a sandwich with whole-wheat bread or sourdough, pay attention to how your stomach and digestive tract react over the next few hours. No problems? Good news—you can indulge in a sub every once in a while. However, if you feel bloated and your energy evaporates, you may want to stick with your gluten-free alternatives to satisfy your sandwich cravings.

And if at any time your weight starts creeping up, you'll want to eliminate the sources of gluten you've added back. The good news is that most people can manage a modified gluten-free eating approach while preserving their weight loss.

Keep Moving

If you're serious about avoiding weight regain, you'll need to stay active. One of the more robust research findings from the field of weight-loss maintenance has been the important role of regular exercise in keeping you slim. A study from the National Weight Control Registry found that people who were able to lose 30 pounds and keep it off for more than a year relied on a combination of diet and exercise; dieters who rely on one or the other aren't nearly as successful.

Lucky for you, you've already found the types of moves that keep you happy and engaged in staying fit; now you just have to be sure to make them a regular part of your life. That will mean staying injury free. One thing that will help is maintaining your strength, so continue to follow the strength-training regimen in Chapter 12. But you may also want to add a flexibility component to your exercise regimen. Regular stretching can keep your ligaments, tendons, and muscles pliable. A simple yoga routine can do wonders for your body, and it will help you release stress, which also plays a role in weight gain.

If you've never done yoga, check out a beginners class in your town or try a DVD at home. You'll soon come to love the way regular stretching feels. It can feel like lubricating your joints—you'll move easier, your performance during exercise will improve, and you'll experience less soreness when you're finished. Just remember to start slowly and go easy on your body. If you've never tried this type of stretching before, you may discover that your joints are nowhere near as flexible as those of the other participants in class or the instructor on your DVD. Don't worry about that, and definitely don't try to mimic or keep up with these people. Listen to your body, and only bend as far as feels comfortable. With time, you'll become much more flexible (although some people never attain the kind of flexibility on display in most yoga classes).

By the way, if you're looking for motivation to keep eating more protein than you once did, a study from a couple of years ago shows that a diet high in protein suits your exercise efforts. Remember the old canard about carb-loading before you exert yourself? Turns out it isn't nearly as effective as protein-loading. Researchers at the University of Stirling in Scotland asked cyclists to follow two identical three-week training sessions. The first week was normal effort, the second week was intensified training, and the third week was a recovery period. During the first session, the cyclists consumed a high-protein diet (about 1.5 grams of protein per pound of bodyweight); during the second session they ate normal meals with normal protein content—about half that of the high-protein diet—and made up the difference with carbohydrates.

On the high-protein regimen, the athletes not only performed better, but they also recovered faster after the intense training sessions. The athletes also reported feeling stronger when they got more protein. In other words, to get the most out of your exercise—and to bring your best effort—eat protein.

Simple Portion Control

Take a look in your cupboard. Those Frisbee-sized dinner plates and helmet-sized cereal bowls aren't doing you or your family any favors. The sad truth is that we eat what's put in front of us, regardless of how much there may be. Brian Wansink, a behavioral psychologist at Cornell University, has tested this in numerous ways. (One of his most devious experiments was a soup bowl that could continuously be filled surreptitiously from the bottom. Sitting around a table, volunteers engaged in conversation would continue to eat as long as there was soup in the bowl, no matter how full they felt.) Wansink has found that reducing your plate size by just 2 inches in diameter can reduce the amount of calories you take in by as much as 25 percent. Choose smaller cereal bowls and you'll get the same effect. Accounting for just breakfast and dinner, you could eliminate 350 calories a day. You could lose a pound every 10 days by doing this alone.

Shop Smart

As you have no doubt come to realize, a grocery list is invaluable when you're following a gluten-free plan. To maintain your loss, you'll want to keep your kitchen well stocked with gluten-free foods. For that reason, you'll always want to go through your kitchen before shopping to replenish any of the staples that are running low.

However, you may also want to start experimenting with new gluten-free foods. When you do, it will be helpful to make sure you understand the various labels on food packaging. Here's a quick guide:

"Low Sodium," "Reduced Sodium"

"Low sodium" means the product has to deliver fewer than 140 milligrams per serving. But "reduced sodium" just means that you're getting 25 percent less than the original item. If a food is extremely high in sodium already, like most canned soups, hitting the reduced-sodium bar is relatively easy. And if a manufacturer is reducing the salt content, it might be jacking up the sugar or fat content to boost flavor.

"Contains Real Fruit"

Sadly, these labels rarely say how much real fruit the food contains. You'll find this kind of label on fruit candy, sugary drinks that seem like orange juice, and other junky foods that are looking for the healthy stamp of approval to help harried moms feel better about buying the snack for children. Do yourself and your family a favor and check the number of sugar grams per serving. Compare brands and choose the item that has the lowest amount of sugar. (Be sure to check the serving size as well. If the package or bottle is something your child would finish in one sitting, but the nutrition label says it contains more than one serving, put it back on the shelf. The manufacturer has split up the servings because this food has too much sugar, fat, or calories in it.) The best way to get your fruit is in its original form, or by juicing it yourself at home. Skip the packaged stuff at the store.

"All Natural"

Food manufacturers trying to jump on the organic bandwagon coined this term. Unfortunately, it's meaningless. Unlike the term "organic," the government has very loose definitions for the term "all natural," and it can be slapped on any number of products that contain not-so-natural ingredients, according to the Center for Science in the Public Interest. The group found that products with the "all natural" labeling included teas sweetened with high-fructose corn syrup, chickens injected with high-sodium broth, and juices with artificial dyes. Don't be fooled by this wording.

Reward Yourself

Let's face it. You're putting in a lot of hard work losing weight and adapting to a new way of eating. So when you shed some pounds, indulge yourself. Shop for some new clothes, or give yourself a night out at a restaurant that can handle your gluten-free needs. Maybe you need a tennis racket or new exercise shoes. Set a weight goal, and when you hit it, give yourself a treat.

A Quick Restart

A great trick to keep your weight in check is keeping a food diary, which will be discussed more in depth in the next chapter. Any time you begin regaining weight, one of the first things you can try is restarting your food diary. This will help you track your gluten-free versus gluten intake. You may discover that you've let several forbidden foods creep back into your meals.

You may also discover that some new stress is pushing you to eat more, such as a new job, money pressures, or troubles with your kids. If emotions are driving you to overdo it, the quickest way to recognize and correct the problem is to use that food diary.

If things really get out of hand, try going through the four-week plan again. You'll quickly shed any pounds you may have regained, and you'll get a refresher course in gluten-free eating.

WHEN YOU'RE LOSING weight or trying to maintain your weight loss, you can't beat a little journaling to help you get a handle on the way you eat. A food diary is a powerful ally in your war on weight.

Studies demonstrate that the food diary is a very consistent and reliable contributor to weight loss. As it turns out, the simple act of writing down what you ate will make you more conscious of your intake and help you avoid overeating. Do it for the first four weeks of the diet and you'll naturally become more conscious of your eating habits and choices.

Keeping a food diary can serve another purpose: divining how much of your eating may be driven by your emotions. That's why there are entries for your mood on the diary pages that follow. Tracking *when* and *why* you eat may be as important to weight loss as tracking what you put on your plate. By cooking more and keeping gluten-free food and snacks around the house you can be sure that, when you eat, you'll choose food that will satisfy you and support your efforts to lose. But you'll also need to rein in urges to eat that are driven by stress, anger, loneliness, and other emotions.

For the next several weeks, keep the following diary pages with you. When you go to grab something to eat, record your emotional state. Are you bored? Are you upset about something that just happened? Are you mulling over a slight from earlier in the day? Then go ahead and eat, but halfway through, stop and make note of how you're feeling after you've had some food.

After a week, flip back through the journal and zero in on the times you saw a distinct improvement in your mood once you began eating. You've identified your emotional eating triggers, and now you can look for ways to replace the urge to eat with a healthier outlet for your feelings. A brisk walk, a phone call to a friend or loved one, taking time for some deep breathing, or simply chewing gum could make a big dent in your calorie intake.

Perhaps one of the most interesting aspects of keeping a food journal while on a gluten-free plan is that you'll find that you're thinking about eating much less than you once did. After a week or two, flip back through your journal and note how your eating habits have changed!

DAY OF WEEK	TIME OF DAY	MEAL

What are you eating?	
How hungry are you?	
Where are you?	
Describe your mood.	

DAY OF WEEK	TIME OF DAY	MEAL

What are you eating?	
How hungry are you?	
Where are you?	
Describe your mood.	

DAY OF WEEK	TIME OF DAY	MEAL

What are you eating?	
How hungry are you?	
Where are you?	
Describe your mood.	

DAY OF WEEK	TIME OF DAY	MEAL

What are you eating?	
How hungry are you?	
Where are you?	
Describe your mood.	

DAY OF WEEK	TIME OF DAY	MEAL

What are you eating?	
How hungry are you?	
Where are you?	
Describe your mood.	

DAY OF WEEK	TIME OF DAY	MEAL

What are you eating?	
How hungry are you?	
Where are you?	
Describe your mood.	

DAY OF WEEK	TIME OF DAY	MEAL

What are you eating?	
How hungry are you?	
Where are you?	
Describe your mood.	

DAY OF WEEK	TIME OF DAY	MEAL

What are you eating?	
How hungry are you?	
Where are you?	
Describe your mood.	

DAY OF WEEK	TIME OF DAY	MEAL

What are you eating?	
How hungry are you?	
Where are you?	
Describe your mood.	

DAY OF WEEK	TIME OF DAY	MEAL

What are you eating?	
How hungry are you?	
Where are you?	
Describe your mood.	

DAY OF WEEK	TIME OF DAY	MEAL

What are you eating?	
How hungry are you?	
Where are you?	
Describe your mood.	

DAY OF WEEK	TIME OF DAY	MEAL

What are you eating?	
How hungry are you?	
Where are you?	
Describe your mood.	

DAY OF WEEK	TIME OF DAY	MEAL

What are you eating?	
How hungry are you?	
Where are you?	
Describe your mood.	

DAY OF WEEK	TIME OF DAY	MEAL

What are you eating?	
How hungry are you?	
Where are you?	
Describe your mood.	

DAY OF WEEK	TIME OF DAY	MEAL

What are you eating?	
How hungry are you?	
Where are you?	
Describe your mood.	

DAY OF WEEK	TIME OF DAY	MEAL

What are you eating?	
How hungry are you?	
Where are you?	
Describe your mood.	

DAY OF WEEK	TIME OF DAY	MEAL

What are you eating?	
How hungry are you?	
Where are you?	
Describe your mood.	

DAY OF WEEK	TIME OF DAY	MEAL

What are you eating?	
How hungry are you?	
Where are you?	
Describe your mood.	

DAY OF WEEK	TIME OF DAY	MEAL

What are you eating?	
How hungry are you?	
Where are you?	
Describe your mood.	

DAY OF WEEK	TIME OF DAY	MEAL

What are you eating?	
How hungry are you?	
Where are you?	
Describe your mood.	

DAY OF WEEK	TIME OF DAY	MEAL
What are you eating?		
How hungry are you?		
Where are you?		
Describe your mood.		

DAY OF WEEK	TIME OF DAY	MEAL
What are you eating?		
How hungry are you?		
Where are you?		
Describe your mood.		

DAY OF WEEK	TIME OF DAY	MEAL
What are you eating?		
How hungry are you?		
Where are you?		
Describe your mood.		

DAY OF WEEK	TIME OF DAY	MEAL
What are you eating?		
How hungry are you?		
Where are you?		
Describe your mood.		

DAY OF WEEK	TIME OF DAY	MEAL

What are you eating?	
How hungry are you?	
Where are you?	
Describe your mood.	

DAY OF WEEK	TIME OF DAY	MEAL

What are you eating?	
How hungry are you?	
Where are you?	
Describe your mood.	

DAY OF WEEK	TIME OF DAY	MEAL

What are you eating?	
How hungry are you?	
Where are you?	
Describe your mood.	

DAY OF WEEK	TIME OF DAY	MEAL

What are you eating?	
How hungry are you?	
Where are you?	
Describe your mood.	

Nutritional Information

HOW TO USE IT AND WHY

The following is a helpful guide to put the nutritional analysis numbers into perspective. Remember, one size doesn't fit all, so take your lifestyle, age, and circumstances into consideration when determining your nutrition needs.

IN OUR NUTRITIONAL ANALYSIS, WE USE THESE ABBREVIATIONS

sat saturated fat	**poly** polyunsaturated fat	**CHOL** cholesterol	**g** gram
mono monounsaturated fat	**CARB** carbohydrates	**CALC** calcium	**mg** milligram

DAILY NUTRITION GUIDE

	Women ages 25 to 50	Women over 50	Men ages 24 to 50	Men over 50
Calories	2,000	2,000 or less	2,700	2,500
Protein	50g	50g or less	63g	60g
Fat	65g or less	65g or less	88g or less	83g or less
Saturated Fat	20g or less	20g or less	27g or less	25g or less
Carbohydrates	304g	304g	410g	375g
Fiber	25g to 35g	25g to 35g	25g to 35g	25g to 35g
Cholesterol	300mg or less	300mg or less	300mg or less	300mg or less
Iron	18mg	8mg	8mg	8mg
Sodium	2,300mg or less	1,500mg or less	2,300mg or less	1,500mg or less
Calcium	1,000mg	1,200mg	1,000mg	1,000mg

The nutritional values used in our calculations either come from The Food Processor, Version 10.4 (ESHA Research), or are provided by food manufacturers.

Metric Equivalents

The information in the following charts is provided to help cooks outside the United States successfully use the recipes in this book. All equivalents are approximate.

COOKING/OVEN TEMPERATURE

Farenheit	225°F	250°F	275°F	300°F	325°F	350°F	375°F	400°F	425°F	450°F	475°F	500°F
Celsius	110°C	120°C	135°C	150°C	160°C	180°C	190°C	205°C	220°C	230°C	245°C	260°C

LENGTH
(To convert inches to centimeters, multiply the number of inches by 2.5.)

1 in = 2.5 cm
6 in = ½ ft = 15 cm
12 in = 1 ft = 30 cm
36 in = 3 ft = 1 yd = 90 cm
40 in = 100 cm = 1 m

LIQUID INGREDIENTS BY VOLUME

1 tsp = 1 ml
3 tsp = 1 Tbsp = ½ fl oz = 15 ml
2 Tbsp = ⅛ cup = 1 fl oz = 30 ml
16 Tbsp = 1 cup = 8 fl oz = 240 ml
1 pt = 2 cups = 16 fl oz = 480 ml
1 qt = 4 cups = 32 fl oz = 960 ml
33 fl oz = 1000 ml = 1 l

DRY INGREDIENTS BY WEIGHT
(To convert ounces to grams, multiply the number of ounces by 30.)

1 oz = 1/16 lb = 30 g
4 oz = ¼ lb = 120 g
8 oz = ½ lb = 240 g
12 oz = ¾ lb = 360 g
16 oz = 1 lb = 480 g

References

CHAPTER 1: GLUTEN FREE AND YOUR HEALTH

Murray JA. *Mayo Clinic Going Gluten Free: Essential Guide to Managing Celiac Disease and Related Conditions.* Birmingham: Oxmoor House. 2014.

Davis JL. The Risks of Belly Fat. WebMD. www.webmd.com

Atkinson SA, Josse AR, Phillips SM, Tarnopolsky MA. Increased consumption of dairy foods and protein during diet- and exercise- induced weight loss promotes fat mass and lean mass gain in overweight and obese premenopausal women. *Journal of Nutrition*. 2011; 141: 1626-1634.

Aller EE, Larsen TM, Claus H, Lindroos AK, Kafatos A, Pheiffer A, Martinez JA, Handjieva-Darlenska T, Kunesova M, Stender S, Saris WH, Astrup A, van Baak MA. Weight loss in overweight subjects on ad libitum diets with high or low protein content and glycemic index: the Diogenes trial 12-month results. *International Journal of Obesity*. 2014; 38: 1511-1517.

Dietary Guidelines for Americans, 2010. www.dietaryguidelines.gov

Voegtlin, WL. *The Stone Age Diet*. New York: Vantage Press, Inc. 1975.

CHAPTER 2: WHY GOING GLUTEN FREE IS GOOD FOR YOU

Cordain L. *The Paleo Diet: Lose Weight and Get Healthy by Eating Foods You Were Designed to Eat.* New Jersey: John Wiley & Sons, Inc. 2002, 2011.

Layman DK, Evans EM, Erickson D, Seyler J, Weber J, Bagshaw D, Griel A, Psota T, Kris-Etherton. A moderate-protein diet produces sustained weight loss and long-term changes in body composition and blood lipids in obese adults. *Journal of Nutrition*. 2009; 139: 514-521

The Paleo Diet. www.thepaleodiet.com

Mark's Daily Apple. www.marksdailyapple.com

CHAPTER 12: EXERCISING FOR GLUTEN-FREE HEALTH

Boutcher SH. High-intensity exercise and fat loss. *Journal of Obesity*. 2011; 2011: 868305

Trapp EG, Chisholm DJ, Freud J, Boutcher SH. The effects of high-intensity intermittent exercise training on fat loss and fasting insulin levels of young women. *International Journal of Obesity*. 2008; 32: 684-691

For All-Day Metabolism Boost, Try Interval Training. American College of Sports Medicine. www.acsm.org

Wycherley TP, Noakes M, Clifton PM, Cleanthous X, Keogh JB, Brinkworth GD. High-Protein Diet with Resistance Exercise Training Improves Weight Loss and Body Composition in Overweight and Obese Patients with Type 2 Diabetes. *Diabetes Care*. 2010; 33: 969-976

When to See a Doctor. American College of Sports Medicine. www.acsm.org

Physical Activity and Health. Centers for Disease Control and Prevention. www.cdc.gov

CHAPTER 13: MAINTAIN YOUR GAINS THE GLUTEN-FREE WAY

Sciamanna CN, Kiernan M, Rolls BJ, Boan J, Stuckey H, Kephart D, Miller CK Practices Associated with Weight Loss Versus Weight-Loss Maintenance. *Preventative Medicine*. 2011; 41: 159-166

Wansink B. Why Visual Cues of Portion Size May Influence Intake. Cornell University Food and Brand Lab. www.foodpsychology.cornell.edu

Index

ISBN-13: 978-0-8487-4483-0
ISBN-10: 0-8487-4483-7
Library of Congress Control Number: 2015933187
Printed in the United States of America
First Printing 2015

Be sure to check with your health-care provider
before making any changes in your diet.

Oxmoor House

Editorial Director: Anja Schmidt
Creative Director: Felicity Keane
Art Director: Christopher Rhoads
Executive Photography Director: Iain Bagwell
Executive Food Director: Grace Parisi
Photo Editor: Kellie Lindsey
Managing Editor: Elizabeth Tyler Austin
Assistant Managing Editor: Jeanne de Lathouder

The 10 Pounds Off Gluten-Free Diet

Senior Editor: Betty Wong
Editor: Rachel Quinlivan West, R.D.
Editorial Assistant: April Smitherman
Assistant Test Kitchen Manager:
    Alyson Moreland Haynes
Recipe Developers and Testers: Julia Levy,
    Stefanie Maloney, Callie Nash, Karen Rankin
Food Stylists: Nathan Carrabba,
    Victoria E. Cox, Margaret Monroe Dickey,
    Catherine Crowell Steele
Senior Photographer: Hélène Dujardin

Senior Photo Stylists: Kay E. Clarke,
    Mindi Shapiro Levine
Production Manager: Theresa Beste-Farley
Assistant Production Director: Sue Chodakiewicz

Contributors

Writer: John Hastings
Assistant Project Editor: Melissa Brown
Designer: Ben Margherita
Junior Designer: AnnaMaria Jacob
Copy Editors: Dolores Hydock,
    *Marra*thon Production Services
Proofreader: Kate Johnson
Indexer: *Marra*thon Production Services
Nutrition Reviewer: Barbara Linhardt, R.D.
Fitness Reviewer: Michele Stanten
Fellows: Laura Arnold, Kylie Dazzo, Nicole Fisher,
    Loren Lorenzo, Anna Ramia, Caroline Smith,
    Amanda Widis

Time Inc. Books

Publisher: Margot Schupf
Vice President, Finance: Vandana Patel
Executive Director, Marketing Services:
    Carol Pittard
Executive Director, Business Development:
    Suzanne Albert
Executive Director, Marketing: Susan Hettleman
Assistant General Counsel: Simone Procas
Assistant Project Manager: Allyson Angle

Photo Credits

Courtesy of: 15 Carmen Kelly, before and
after; 39 Dorothy Herbst, before and after **Getty
Images:** 6, 10, 20, 28, 42, 50, 62, 66, 86, 106,
144, 164, 188, 202, 210 DNY59, scale; 34 Alasdair
Thomson, buckwheat; 37 Kadir Barcin, rice

Back cover

Left: Sautéed Tilapia Tacos with Grilled Peppers
    and Onion, page 114
Right: Shredded Chicken Tacos with Tomatoes
    and Grilled Corn, page 127

The
TOP 100
CAJUN
RECIPES
of all time

Edited by
Trent Angers

Acadian House
PUBLISHING
Lafayette, Louisiana

Library of Congress Cataloging-in-Publication Data

The Top 100 cajun recipes of all time / edited by Trent M. Angers.
    p. cm.
  Includes index.
  ISBN 0-925417-52-1
1. Cookery, American—Louisiana style. 2. Cookery, Cajun.
I. Angers, Trent.
  TX715.2.L68T66 2005
  641.59763—dc22

          2005019402

- ♦ **Published by Acadian House Publishing, Lafayette, Louisiana. (Edited by Trent Angers; interior graphic design and production by Jon Russo.)**

- ♦ **Cover design by Tom Sommers, Crowley, Louisiana**

- ♦ **Printed by Walsworth Printing, Marceline, Missouri, USA**

PREFACE

The Cradle Of Cajun Cooking

Cajun cooking originated in south Louisiana a couple of centuries ago when the French-Acadians (known today by many as "Cajuns") first settled this land after being exiled, for political reasons, from what is known today as Nova Scotia.

In the years since, Cajun cooking has been developed into something of an art form in the kitchens of south Louisiana – specifically in the 22-parish region called Acadiana, or "Cajun country."

For the record, this area is composed of the parishes of Acadia, Ascension, Assumption, Avoyelles, Calcasieu, Cameron, Evangeline, Iberia, Iberville, Jefferson Davis, Lafayette, Lafourche, Pointe Coupee, St. Charles, St. James, St. John the Baptist, St. Landry, St. Martin, St. Mary, Terrebonne, Vermilion and West Baton Rouge. (For a more detailed map, please turn the page.)

The people of this region are proud of their accomplishments in the culinary field and are pleased to share their brand of cooking with others around the world.

– *T.A.*

The 22 parishes of Acadiana, or 'Cajun Country'

The Cream of the Crop Of Cajun Recipes

Cajun cooking today is one of America's most exciting and delicious kinds of cooking. Over the past 30 years, its reputation has spread throughout the United States.

This is due in part to the inherent goodness of Cajun food, to a tremendous amount of newspaper, magazine and TV publicity, and to the dozens of cookbooks that feature Cajun recipes.

Some of these cookbooks were published by our company, Acadian House Publishing, and its affiliate, *Acadiana Profile* Magazine. Now, after decades of experience in the business, we have compiled this cookbook containing what we consider to be some of the best Cajun recipes in existence today. We think of them as the cream of the crop of Cajun recipes. (By the way, the softcover version of this book was first published in 1995. This hardcover edition is a companion to the hardcover of *The Top 100 NEW ORLEANS Recipes Of All Time.*)

The recipes in the book you are holding were selected mostly from our best-selling *Cajun Cooking Cookbooks (Parts 1 & 2), The Louisiana Gumbo Cookbook, The Louisiana Festivals Cookbook,* and from special recipe editions of *Acadiana Profile*, "The Magazine of the Cajun Country."

The recipe-selection process was rather involved. But, to make a long story short, we tried to include recipes for the real classics of

Cajun cooking, those recipes that are readily recognizable as coming from south Louisiana. For instance, crawfish *etouffee,* chicken *fricassee, couche couche, boudin, maque choux, sauce piquante,* and catfish *courtbouillon.*

We also made an effort to include recipes that would help to balance the diet, even though they might not be considered by some to be among the classics of Cajun cuisine. For example, smothered okra and eggplant, candied yams, potato salad, and "dirty rice."

And we added a group of sweets that may not be good for the waistline but are certainly good for one's disposition! Such as pralines, pecan pie, rice pudding and blackberry dumplings...

In the process of selecting these recipes, we reached one conclusion of which we are fairly certain: Most of the recipes contained in this book have contributed in a real way to south Louisiana's well-deserved reputation for having some of the best food in the United States, if not the entire world.

– Trent Angers
Editor

TABLE OF CONTENTS

Two Basic Recipes Important in Cajun Cooking

R<small>OUX</small>

- 4 tablespoons of oil
- 6 tablespoons of flour

1. Heat oil in pot; add flour, stirring constantly over medium-high heat until brown.

2. Lower heat and continue cooking and stirring until dark brown.

Some of the recipes in this cookbook vary, but these are the basic proportions of oil to flour. Specific quantities differ with the different recipes, of course.

R<small>ICE</small>

- 1 cup of rice
- 2 cups of water
- 1 tablespoon of oil or butter
- 1 teaspoon of salt

1. Put all ingredients in a two-quart saucepan and bring to a boil.

2. Lower heat to medium and cook until rice and water are at the same level.

3. Cover, lower heat to low, and cook 20 minutes.

4. Remove from heat and let stand for five to ten minutes before serving.

Another way to measure the proportions of rice to water is to add enough water to the pan to cover the rice by the depth of one finger joint (index finger). This rule applies no matter how much rice you're cooking.

The TOP 100 CAJUN RECIPES of all time

The Evangeline Oak in downtown St. Martinville is said to be the tree under which the heroine of Longfellow's poem, "Evangeline," arrived by boat upon completion of her journey from Nova Scotia after being exiled along with her fellow Acadians.

CRAB-STUFFED MIRLITON

- ❏ 4 to 5 mirlitons
- ❏ 1 large onion, finely chopped
- ❏ Cooking oil
- ❏ ½ cup of chopped parsley
- ❏ 1 cup of chopped green onions
- ❏ ½ stalk of celery, chopped
- ❏ 1 large bellpepper, chopped
- ❏ Salt and pepper, to taste
- ❏ 1 cup of cooked rice
- ❏ 1 pound of crabmeat
- ❏ Breadcrumbs

1. Boil mirlitons until tender; cut off tops; scoop-out inside pulp, leaving shells intact to stuff later.

2. Sauté onion in oil in skillet.

3. Add mirliton pulp; cook until tender.

4. Combine parsley, green onions, celery, bellpepper, salt, pepper and rice; add to sautéed vegetables; add crabmeat; mix.

5. Stuff into mirliton shells; top with breadcrumbs.

6. Bake uncovered in casserole at 350 degrees for about 30 minutes.

– Susan Guilbeau
Lafayette (Lafayette Parish)

*B*OUDIN

- ❑ 2 pounds of pork meat
- ❑ 1½ pounds of pork liver
- ❑ Salt and pepper, to taste
- ❑ 1 large onion, cut up
- ❑ 2 bunches of green onions, chopped
- ❑ 1 bunch of parsley, chopped
- ❑ 6 cups of cooked rice
- ❑ Sausage casings, soaked in cold water

1. Cook pork meat, liver and seasonings in water to cover until meat falls apart; remove meat and reserve some broth.

2. Grind meat, onion, green onions and parsley (reserving about one-half cup each of green onion tops and parsley).

3. Mix ground meat mixture with the one-half cups of green onion and parsley, rice and enough broth to make a moist dressing.

4. Stuff dressing into casings, using a sausage-stuffer.

– Sue C. McDonough
New Iberia (Iberia Parish)

Paté de Fois Gras
(Liver Paté)

- ☐ 4 pounds of pork livers
- ☐ 3 pounds of pork meat
- ☐ 2 pounds of pork fat
- ☐ 7 small garlic cloves, minced
- ☐ 3 tablespoons of salt
- ☐ 4 teaspoons of black pepper
- ☐ 1 tablespoon of red pepper

1. Grind liver, meat and fat together twice; mix well and place in a large pot.

2. Add garlic, seasonings and water to cover (about four and three-fourths cups).

3. Cook until fat rises to the top (about three hours), stirring often.

4. Pour in jars; refrigerate. (The fat will rise to the top of the jar; this acts as a seal.)

5. Before serving, bring to room temperature; with a fork, work the fat back into the paté. (This makes it easier to spread).

6. Serve with crackers or French bread.

– Mrs. Sam Broussard
New Iberia (Iberia Parish)

CRABMEAT DIP

- ❑ 2 cups of crabmeat
- ❑ 1-8 ounce can of water chestnuts, drained and chopped
- ❑ 2 tablespoons of soy sauce
- ❑ ½ cup of mayonnaise
- ❑ 1 tablespoon of chopped fresh ginger root (ground ginger may be substituted)
- ❑ 6 to 8 crab claws for garnish (optional)
- ❑ Bread sticks (for serving)
- ❑ Celery sticks (for serving)

1. Combine all the ingredients except the last three.

2. Pile in serving bowl and chill; garnish with crab claws. Serve bread sticks or celery sticks for dipping.

– Mrs. Jerry Jones
Cameron (Cameron Parish)

*H*OG'S HEAD CHEESE

- ❑ 1 fresh pork picnic ham with skin
- ❑ 7 shallots, chopped
- ❑ 1 cup of parsley, chopped
- ❑ Paprika (for coloring)
- ❑ 6 fresh pork hocks or pig feet
- ❑ 4 garlic cloves, chopped
- ❑ Red pepper and salt, to taste

1. Simmer all ingredients in a large pot with enough water to cover meat; cook until tender.

2. Remove from broth and cool; chop meat and skin into small pieces. Discard fat.

3. Return meat to broth and simmer until thick.

4. Pour into loaf pans and cool. Refrigerate.

– Myrtle Millet
Reserve (St. John the Baptist Parish)

Docked on a bayou near Houma, these shrimp boats are part of the fleet that works in the Gulf of Mexico to harvest one of Louisiana's most popular foods.

*C*ANDIED YAMS

- ❑ 6 or 7 medium yams
- ❑ ½ cup of sugar
- ❑ 1 cup of white corn syrup
- ❑ ¼ teaspoon of salt
- ❑ 2 tablespoons of butter

1. Boil yams until tender; peel and place cut yams in buttered dish.

2. Heat sugar, corn syrup, salt and butter; pour over yams.

3. Bake at 425 degrees for 45 to 60 minutes. Turn over often.

– Germaine Porta
Gramercy (St. James Parish)

*M*AQUE CHOUX

- ❑ 24 ears of sweet corn
- ❑ 2 onions, finely chopped
- ❑ 2 large bellpeppers, chopped
- ❑ 4 over-sized tomatoes, or 1 15-ounce can of whole tomatoes
- ❑ ½ pound of butter
- ❑ 2 tablespoons of salt
- ❑ 2 tablespoons of black pepper

1. Cut corn off the cob; shave down the cob to get the juice. (Shave each cob right after cutting kernels from it; then move on to the next.)

2. Sauté onion, bellpepper and tomato in butter for about 10 minutes.

3. Add corn and cook until tender, about 15 minutes. (If corn takes longer to get soft, add some milk and a little more butter.)

4. Add salt and pepper about five minutes into cooking corn.

– Alex Patout
New Iberia (Iberia Parish)

"DIRTY RICE"

- ❏ 1 bunch of green onions, chopped
- ❏ ½ bellpepper, chopped
- ❏ 2 ribs of celery, chopped
- ❏ ½ pound of chicken livers and gizzards, mixed
- ❏ ½ pound of calf's liver
- ❏ ¼ pound of ground beef
- ❏ 3 tablespoons of oil
- ❏ Salt and pepper, to taste
- ❏ 3 cups of cooked rice
- ❏ 1 tablespoon of dry parsley
- ❏ 1 tablespoon of chives

1. Grind vegetables and meats.

2. Put oil in a heavy pot with lid. Add ground vegetables and meats. Cover pot. Simmer on low heat one and one-half hours. Season, to taste.

3. Mix rice and vegetable-meat mixture. Stir thoroughly. Add dry parsley and chives.

– Mr. Teska Moreau
Marksville (Avoyelles Parish)

*B*UTTERBEANS WITH *R*OUX

- ❑ 1 tablespoon of flour
- ❑ 2 tablespoons of oil
- ❑ 1 small onion, chopped
- ❑ 1 pound of fresh butterbeans
- ❑ 1 quart of water
- ❑ Salt and pepper, to taste
- ❑ 1 tablespoon of sugar (optional)

1. Brown flour in oil to make the roux; add onion and butterbeans and cook lightly.

2. Add water and cook until beans are tender and gravy is thick. Salt and pepper, to taste. Add sugar if desired.

– Mrs. Louis Courtade, Sr.
Brusly (West Baton Rouge Parish)

Smothered Eggplant

- ❑ 1 stick of butter
- ❑ 2 large onions, chopped
- ❑ 1 bellpepper, chopped
- ❑ 3 fresh tomatoes, sliced
- ❑ 1 large eggplant, sliced ¾-inch thick
  and soaked in cold salted water
- ❑ 2 garlic cloves, mashed
- ❑ 1 teaspoon of salt
- ❑ ½ teaspoon of Tabasco

1. Melt butter over slow heat, sauté onions and bellpepper.

2. Add tomatoes; cook very slowly for about 20 minutes; stir occasionally.

3. Add eggplant, garlic, salt and hot sauce; cover and steam for about 30 minutes.

– Mrs. Alma Phillips
Port Allen (West Baton Rouge Parish)

$\mathcal{S}$MOTHERED OKRA

- ❑ 10 pounds of okra
- ❑ Cooking oil
- ❑ 2 large bellpeppers, chopped
- ❑ 2 large onions, chopped
- ❑ 2 large cans of tomatoes
  (or 4 fresh tomatoes, peeled)
- ❑ Salt and red pepper, to taste

1. Wash okra and slice into one-half inch slices.

2. Pour oil to cover bottom of large heavy roasting pan; add okra, bellpepper and onion, and blend. Cover tightly and cook in 300-degree oven for one hour.

3. Add tomatoes and stir until well-blended; re-cover and continue to cook for at least two more hours. Stir occasionally to prevent sticking.

4. When cooked, add seasonings to taste and serve hot as a side dish, or freeze for later use in gumbo.

– Kathryn Leonard
Lafayette (Lafayette Parish)

*P*OTATO SALAD

- ❑ 8 to 10 small whole red new potatoes
- ❑ 1 hard-cooked egg
- ❑ 2½ cup of mayonnaise
- ❑ 1 tablespoon of lemon juice
- ❑ ¼ cup of half-and-half cream
- ❑ ½ cup of minced green onions
- ❑ ½ cup of minced sweet cucumber pickle slices
- ❑ ¼ cup of minced bellpepper
- ❑ 1 tablespoon of minced parsley
- ❑ 1 teaspoon of salt
- ❑ ½ teaspoon of dill weed
- ❑ ¼ teaspoon of marjoram
- ❑ ½ teaspoon of summer savory
- ❑ ¼ teaspoon of pepper

1. In a large saucepan, boil unpeeled potatoes until fork-tender, for about 20 minutes.

2. In medium bowl, mash the egg thoroughly; stir-in remaining ingredients until well-mixed.

3. Taste for flavor; the dressing may taste salty, but do not be concerned, as the potatoes will absorb the salt.

4. After potatoes are cooked, drain; plunge into cold water and drain immediately.

5. Peel and slice into medium bowl; pour dressing over warm potatoes and toss until well-coated.

6. Cool; then cover and refrigerate until chilled.

Makes four to six servings.

– Mrs. Charles A. Rogers
Cameron (Cameron Parish)

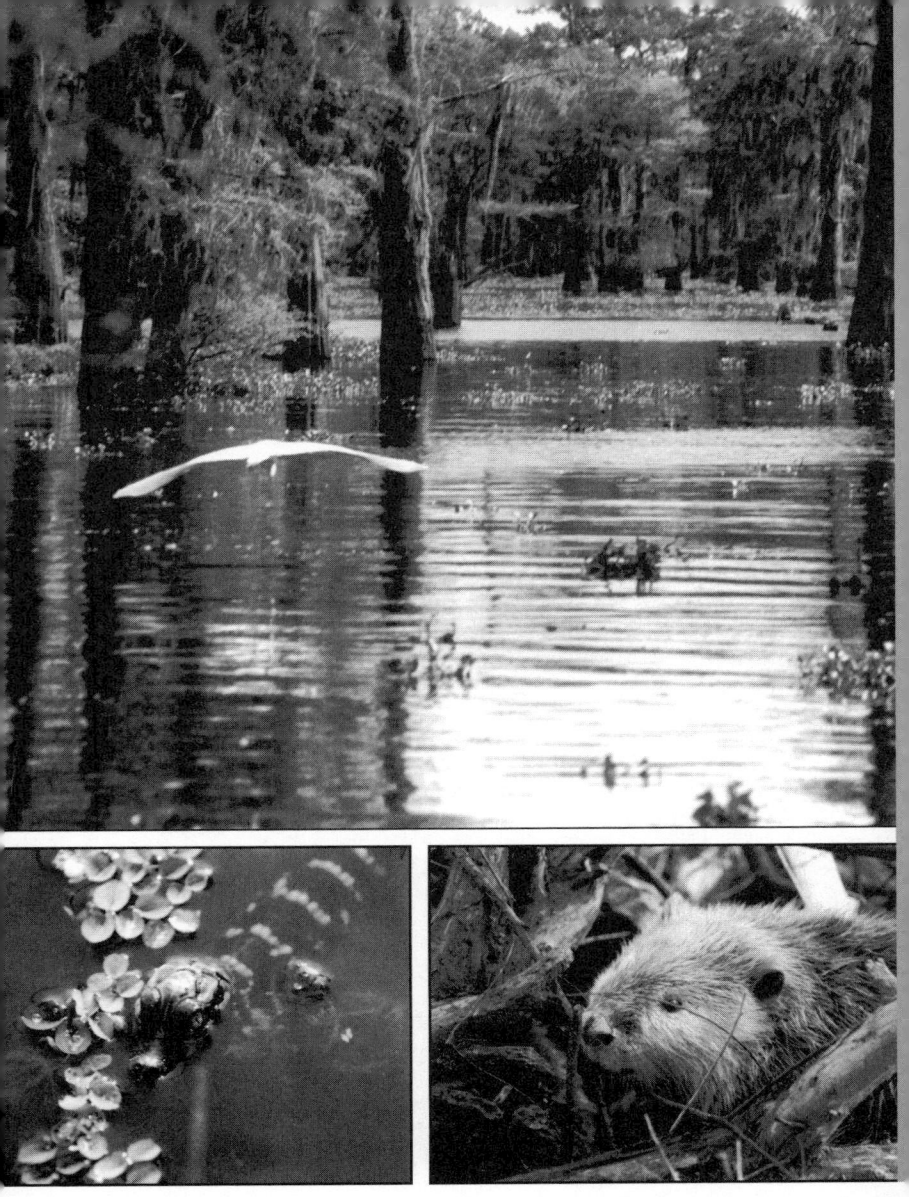

The Atchafalaya River Basin in south-central Louisiana is a vast swampland semi-wilderness area filled with all sorts of furry, feathered and scaly animals.

Turtle Soup

- ❑ 2 pounds of turtle meat, chopped
- ❑ Salt and pepper, to taste
- ❑ 3 tablespoons of oil
- ❑ 3 tablespoons of flour
- ❑ 2 large onions, chopped
- ❑ 1 cup of chopped celery
- ❑ ½ cup of chopped bellpepper
- ❑ 2 garlic cloves, minced
- ❑ 1 cup of tomato sauce
- ❑ Water
- ❑ ½ lemon, sliced
- ❑ 4 bay leaves
- ❑ Parsley
- ❑ ½ cup of sherry
- ❑ 1 tablespoon of Worcestershire sauce
- ❑ 3 hard-cooked eggs

1. Season turtle meat with salt and pepper; fry in oil until brown. Remove from oil. Add flour, browning slowly until golden.

2. Add onions, celery, bellpepper and garlic; cook until tender.

3. Return turtle meat to the pot; add tomato sauce and one cup of water; cook about 30 minutes.

4. Add lemon, bay leaves and two quarts of water; simmer for one hour or until soup has reduced to desired thickness.

5. Add parsley, sherry and Worcestershire sauce.

6. Place slices of hard-cooked eggs (sprinkled with paprika) on soup plates before serving.

Serves six.

– Mrs. Edward Hebert, Jr.
Thibodaux (Lafourche Parish)

CHICKEN & SAUSAGE GUMBO

- ❑ 2 cups of flour
- ❑ 1¾ cups of oil
- ❑ 1 large onion, chopped
- ❑ 2 stalks of celery, chopped
- ❑ 4 quarts of water
- ❑ 1 large hen, cut into serving pieces
  (Don't use a fryer)
- ❑ 3 to 5 pounds of sausage,
  cut into 2-inch pieces
- ❑ 1 bunch of onion tops, chopped
- ❑ 4 or 5 stalks of parsley, chopped

1. Stir flour in oil on medium-high heat to make a roux. Cook until the roux reaches the color of dark coffee.

2. Add chopped onion and celery. Stir for a short period.

3. Add four quarts of water and chicken.

4. Boil one hour, adding salt and pepper, to taste.

5. Add sausage and boil another hour.

6. Skim fat off top.

7. Add onion tops and parsley.

8. Serve over rice in soup plates.

Makes 12 to 14 servings.

– Marie L. Broussard
Kaplan (Vermilion Parish)

REDFISH COURTBOUILLON

- ❑ 1 cup of flour
- ❑ ¾ cup of oil
- ❑ 1 cup of chopped onion
- ❑ 1 medium bellpepper, chopped fine
- ❑ 2 cans of tomato paste
- ❑ 1 can of stewed tomatoes
- ❑ 3 garlic cloves, minced
- ❑ 1 cup of chopped celery
- ❑ 1 lemon, sliced thin
- ❑ 2 bay leaves
- ❑ Salt and pepper, to taste
- ❑ 4 to 6 pounds of de-boned fish (leave skin on for better taste)
- ❑ 12 sprigs of parsley, chopped fine
- ❑ 1 tablespoon of Worcestershire sauce
- ❑ 1 to 2 cups of sauterne wine
- ❑ 2 cans of chopped mushrooms
- ❑ ½ cup of chopped olives

1. Make a dark brown roux with flour and oil. Add onion and bellpepper; stir and cook until vegetables are well-smothered.

2. Add tomato paste and stewed tomatoes; cook thoroughly.

3. Add garlic, celery, lemon slices and bay leaves; season with salt and pepper. Add hot water, a little at a time, up to about four cups; simmer about 15 minutes.

4. Add fish; cook 30 minutes after boiling begins.

5. Add parsley, Worcestershire sauce, wine, mushrooms and olives; bring to a boil and cook for five minutes. Turn off heat and let stand with cover on for a few minutes.

Serve with rice.

– Mrs. S.E. Curole
Larose (Lafourche Parish)

*C*ATFISH *C*OURTBOUILLON

- ❑ 2 tablespoons of butter
- ❑ 2 cups of chopped onion
- ❑ 1 cup of chopped celery
- ❑ 1 cup of chopped bellpepper
- ❑ 1 tablespoon of catsup
- ❑ 1 small can of tomato paste
- ❑ 3 cloves of garlic, minced
- ❑ 1¼ sliced lemons
- ❑ Salt and pepper, to taste
- ❑ Pickled peppers
- ❑ 4 pounds of catfish

1. In butter, sauté onion, celery and bellpepper; add catsup, tomato paste, garlic and lemon.

2. Simmer for three hours on low heat; add salt, pepper and pickled peppers as needed.

3. Add catfish and simmer for 20 minutes. Do not stir after catfish has been added.

– Una Guidry
Lake Arthur (Jefferson Davis Parish)

*S*HRIMP & *O*KRA *G*UMBO

- ❑ 1 quart of okra, cut up
- ❑ 1 medium onion, chopped
- ❑ 1 small bellpepper, chopped
- ❑ 3 ripe tomatoes, peeled and chopped
- ❑ 1 tablespoon of oil
- ❑ 1 teaspoon of salt
- ❑ Pinch of black pepper
- ❑ 1 cup of shrimp peeled
- ❑ 1 quart of water

1. Smother okra with onion, bellpepper, tomatoes and oil.

2. Add salt, pepper, shrimp and water. Cook on low heat for 45 minutes.

Note: Don't use iron pot for cooking okra: it will cause okra to turn black.

– Mrs. Malcolm Guillot
Avoyelles Parish

SHRIMP & OYSTER GUMBO

- ❏ Salt, cayenne pepper and black pepper, to taste
- ❏ 2 pounds of peeled, deveined shrimp
- ❏ ½ cup of fat or cooking oil
- ❏ ¾ cup of all-purpose flour
- ❏ 2 large onions, chopped
- ❏ 1 can of tomatoes, sieved
- ❏ 1 can of tomato paste
- ❏ ¼ cup of bellpepper, chopped
- ❏ 1 cup of chopped celery
- ❏ 2 cloves of garlic, minced
- ❏ 4 quarts of water
- ❏ 1 bottle of clam juice
- ❏ 1 bouillon cube
- ❏ 1½ teaspoons of thyme
- ❏ 1 pound of okra, sliced
- ❏ 1 bay leaf
- ❏ ¾ cup of chopped, cooked ham (6 ounces)
- ❏ 1 pint of oysters, with liquid
- ❏ ½ cup of finely chopped parsley
- ❏ ½ cup of finely chopped green onion tops
- ❏ 6 drops of Tabasco
- ❏ Filé powder

1. In a bowl, combine salt, black pepper and cayenne. Dredge the shrimp in this seasoning mix. Shake off any excess and set the shrimp aside.

2. In a Dutch oven or heavy skillet, heat the fat or cooking oil over medium heat until it is hot. Add the flour gradually in small amounts to make a roux. Stir continuously to avoid burning the roux.

3. Add the onions, tomatoes, tomato paste, bellpepper, celery and garlic. Sauté, stirring occasionally, until the onions appear transparent, about five minutes.

4. Add water, clam juice, bouillon cube, thyme, okra, bay leaf; increase the heat to high and bring to a boil, stirring frequently. Reduce the heat to medium-low and simmer for one hour.

5. Add the shrimp and ham and cook over medium to low heat in uncovered pot for 20 minutes.

6. Add oysters and their liquid and cook until the oyster edges curl.

7. Add parsley and green onion tops.

8. Adjust seasonings to taste, using salt, cayenne pepper, black pepper and Tabasco. Remove bay leaf and discard.

9. To serve, mound rice in preheated gumbo bowls; ladle some gumbo over the rice; garnish with parsley and green onion tops. Each serving should include shrimp, oyster, and ham.

10. Offer filé at the table.

– Bea Weber
Abbeville (Vermilion Parish)

*W*ILD DUCK & OYSTER GUMBO

- ❏ 1 heaping tablespoon of shortening
- ❏ 2 heaping tablespoons of flour
- ❏ 1 large or 2 small onions, chopped
- ❏ 1 wild duck, cut into six pieces
- ❏ Salt and pepper
- ❏ 2 quarts of water
- ❏ 2 dozen oysters and liquid

1. Melt shortening. When hot, add flour to make a roux. When roux is browned, add onion. Cook until tender.

2. Season duck with salt and pepper.

3. When onions are tender in roux, add the duck pieces. Let fry in the roux until blood in duck disappears.

4. Add water. Let boil slowly until duck is very tender.

5. Add oyster liquid and oysters. Cook about ten minutes longer.

6. Season again if necessary after oysters have been added.

– Mrs. Elton Beaullieu
Jeanerette (Iberia Parish)

*O*PELOUSAS OYSTER GUMBO

- ☐ ¼ cup of all-purpose flour
- ☐ ¼ cup of butter or margarine
- ☐ 1 cup of chopped bellpepper
- ☐ 1 cup of chopped onion
- ☐ 1 clove of garlic, crushed
- ☐ 2 cups of water
- ☐ 2 tablespoons of snipped fresh parsley
- ☐ 1 teaspoon of salt
- ☐ ¼ teaspoon each of ground black pepper and dried thyme
- ☐ Dash of ground red pepper
- ☐ 1 bay leaf
- ☐ ½ pound of peeled, deveined raw shrimp
- ☐ 1 pint of oysters with liquid
- ☐ Gumbo filé*
- ☐ 3 cups of hot cooked rice

1. Brown flour in butter until it is a deep red-brown, stirring constantly to prevent burning.

2. Add bellpeppers, onion and garlic. Cook until tender.

3. Stir-in water, parsley and seasonings. Cook slowly for 30 minutes.

4. Add shrimp and oysters with liquid. Bring to a boil and cook five minutes longer, until shrimp are pink and oysters begin to curl.

5. Remove from heat and add gumbo filé, to taste.

6. Serve in shallow bowls over fluffy rice.

*Never add filé while gumbo is cooking, because boiling after filé is added tends to make gumbo stringy.

– USA Rice Council

DUCK GUMBO

- ❑ 6 ducks
- ❑ Creole seasonings, to taste
- ❑ 6 onions, chopped
- ❑ ½ stalk of chopped celery
- ❑ 3 bellpeppers, chopped
- ❑ 1 gallon of water
- ❑ 1 bunch of onion tops, chopped
- ❑ 1 bunch of parsley, chopped

1. Cut up, season and brown ducks.

2. Add chopped onion, celery and bellpepper, then brown ducks more.

3. Add water to mixture and simmer until ducks are tender, about three hours.

4. Add onion tops and parsley; cook an additional 20 minutes.

Serve with rice and baked sweet potatoes.

Serves six to eight.

– Shirley Bonsall
Grand Chenier (Cameron Parish)

*S*EAFOOD *G*UMBO

- ❑ 1 cup of chopped onion
- ❑ ½ cup of chopped bellpepper
- ❑ ½ cup of chopped celery
- ❑ 2 gallons of shrimp stock
- ❑ 1½ cups of roux
- ❑ Salt, cayenne pepper and garlic, to taste
- ❑ 1 pound of medium shrimp, peeled
- ❑ 1 pound of claw crabmeat
- ❑ 1 pint of oysters with juice

1. Combine all ingredients except seafood in a large pot; boil on medium heat until roux is dissolved.

2. Lower heat to a simmer for an additional hour and a half with the pot covered, allowing some steam to escape.

3. For the final minutes of cooking, bring the mixture to a heavy boil, add the seafood ingredients and cook for three minutes, until shrimp are pink.

– Don's Seafood Hut
Lafayette (Lafayette Parish)

*B*LACK'S OYSTER BAR GUMBO

This recipe from Abbeville's famous Black's Oyster Bar will feed a crowd or stock your freezer for the winter.

- ❑ 2 pints of Mazola Corn Oil
- ❑ 3 pints of flour
- ❑ 1 tablespoon of tomato paste
- ❑ 3¼ pounds of onions, diced
- ❑ 3¼ pounds of celery, diced
- ❑ 3½ gallons of oyster liquid, divided
- ❑ 1 teaspoon of Worcestershire
- ❑ 3 tablespoons of Louisiana Hot Sauce
- ❑ 1 tablespoon of Tabasco sauce
- ❑ 1 tablespoon of white pepper
- ❑ 1 tablespoon of black pepper
- ❑ 1 tablespoon of red pepper
- ❑ ½ cup of salt
- ❑ 3 quarts of peeled shrimp, divided
  (Reserve heads and shells.)
- ❑ 2½ gallons of shrimp stock
- ❑ 1 pint of chopped bellpepper
- ❑ Rind of 3 lemons
- ❑ 3 quarts of oysters, divided
- ❑ 4½ pounds of claw crabmeat, divided
- ❑ Green onion tops, chopped

1. In a large Magnalite roasting pan, heat oil on the highest heat possible until the oil smokes. Do not burn the oil. Add the flour. (Enough flour should be added so that when a spoon is drawn through the mixture, the flour appears to follow behind the spoon in its wake.) Constantly stir the roux until it is dark brown. Add the tomato paste.

2. To the roux add the onion and celery. Add two gallons of oyster liquid. (Use the remaining oyster liquid throughout preparation to maintain the liquid volume.) Simmer for five minutes.

3. Add the Worcestershire sauce, Louisiana Hot Sauce, Tabasco, white pepper, black pepper, red pepper and salt. Simmer one and one-half hours, stirring occasionally.

4. Add the reserved shrimp heads and shells to two and one-half gallons of water. Simmer for one-half hour.

5. Strain the shrimp stock and add it to the gumbo. Add additional oyster liquid as needed. Cook for one and one-half hours on medium heat.

6. Add the chopped bellpepper. Cook for another 30 minutes.

7. Add the lemon rinds. Cook for 30 minutes.

8. Divide the six gallons of gumbo into three two-gallon containers and cool. Refrigerate or freeze until ready to serve.

9. To serve, add to one of the two-gallon containers one quart of oysters, one quart of shrimp and one and one-half pounds of claw crabmeat. Simmer for 15 minutes.

10. Serve immediately over hot cooked rice, or refrigerate until needed and reheat in a microwave oven until steaming. (A cup serving should contain two oysters and three shrimp. A bowl should have five oysters and five shrimp.)

11. Garnish each serving with onion tops.

Note: Delicious with potato salad!

Makes six gallons.

– Bryan Bourque
Black's Oyster Bar
Abbeville (Vermilion Parish)

CRAWFISH BISQUE

- 20 pounds of live crawfish
- 6 tablespoons of butter or oleo
- ½ cup of oil
- 1 cup of flour
- 2 large onions, ground
- 1 large bellpepper, ground
- 4½ cups of water
- 1 tablespoon of salt
- 2 teaspoons of red pepper
- ½ cup of chopped green onion tops
- ½ cup of chopped parsley
- Stuffed Crawfish Heads (Recipe follows)

1. Drop live crawfish in boiling water for 10 minutes or until crawfish are red.

2. Separate heads from tails; peel tails and set aside. Place crawfish "fat" in separate container and set aside. Clean 60 heads to fill with stuffing; set aside. Divide tails and "fat" equally for bisque and for stuffing.

3. Make a roux with butter, oil and flour; add onions and bellpepper. Cool until soft, stirring frequently.

4. Add one-half of the crawfish tails and one-half of the crawfish "fat;" cook over low heat for about 20 minutes.

5. Gradually add four and one-half cups of boiling water, salt and pepper; cook for about 20 minutes more.

6. Add onion tops and parsley. Just before serving, add baked Stuffed Crawfish Heads.

Serve with rice.

Serves 10.

STUFFED CRAWFISH HEADS

- ¼ cup of oil
- ½ cup of flour
- 2 medium onions, ground
- 1 large bellpepper, ground
- ¾ cup of water
- 2 teaspoons of salt
- 1½ teaspoons of red pepper
- 1½ cups of breadcrumbs
- ¼ cup of chopped parsley
- ¼ cup of chopped green onion tops
- 4 tablespoons of butter or oleo
- 60 cleaned crawfish heads
- Flour

1. Make a roux with oil and flour; add onions and bellpepper. Cook until soft.

2. Grind remaining crawfish tails and add to onion mixture; add remaining crawfish "fat" and simmer for 15 minutes.

3. Add water, salt, pepper, breadcrumbs, parsley, green onion tops and butter; mix well.

4. Fill each head with stuffing, roll in flour and bake at 350 degrees for 15 minutes.

– Mrs. August Girard
Breaux Bridge (St. Martin Parish)

Gumbo Z'Herbes

- ❑ 1 bunch of fresh spinach greens
- ❑ 1 bunch of fresh turnip greens
- ❑ 1 bunch of fresh mustard greens
- ❑ 1 bunch of fresh collard greens
- ❑ 1 pound of boiled ham, cut into large cubes
- ❑ 1 pound of andouille sausage, cut into large pieces
- ❑ 1 pound of salt meat, cut into large cubes
- ❑ 10 cups of water
- ❑ ½ handful of bay leaves
- ❑ ½ teaspoon of thyme
- ❑ ½ teaspoon of allspice
- ❑ ½ teaspoon of mace
- ❑ Salt and pepper, to taste
- ❑ 1 bunch of fresh parsley
- ❑ 1 cup of chopped celery
- ❑ 1 cup of chopped bellpepper
- ❑ ½ pound of slab bacon, cut in large pieces
- ❑ 2 jumbo onions, chopped
- ❑ ½ stick of butter
- ❑ ½ cup of flour

1. Wash greens very thoroughly several times. Set aside.

2. Place ham, sausage and salt meat into boiling water. Add all seasonings and cook on a rolling boil for about one hour.

3. Strain liquid through a triple-fold cheese cloth and reserve the meat.

4. Dice the salt meat, ham and sausage.

5. Place liquid back on heat and add all greens and vegetables except onions. Cook at a rolling boil for one to one and a half hours.

6. Remove half of the greens from the liquid and chop them coarsely.

7. Sauté bacon until crisp and reserve the grease.

8. Place all cooked ingredients back in the pot. Simmer at low heat.

9. Sauté the onions in butter and one-fourth cup of bacon grease; add flour to make a paste.

10. Add paste to the gumbo and allow it to thicken.

11. Once again, season the gumbo with thyme, mace, allspice salt and pepper. Because of the mild flavor of the greens, you may also want to add a little Accent.

– Yellow Bowl Restaurant
Jeanerette

CORN CHOWDER

- ❑ 4 ears of corn (or 1 pint of frozen cream-style corn)
- ❑ 2 small onions, chopped
- ❑ 2 small green peppers, chopped
- ❑ 4 tablespoons of oleo or butter
- ❑ Flour
- ❑ 1 quart of milk
- ❑ 4 fresh tomatoes, peeled and chopped (or 1 can of tomatoes, drained)
- ❑ Salt and pepper, to taste
- ❑ 1 cup of coffee cream
- ❑ 2 tablespoons of butter

1. Scrape corn from cob; sauté with onions and green peppers in oleo for five minutes, stirring constantly.

2. Sprinkle with a small amount of flour; mix until smooth. Add milk, tomatoes and seasonings, simmer 30 minutes, stirring often.

3. If mixture has a tendency to curdle, add a pinch of soda and stir.

4. When ready to serve, add cream and butter.

Serves six to eight.

– Mrs. Jerry Jones
Cameron (Cameron Parish)

CHICKEN GUMBO

- ❑ 3- to 4-pound fryer, cut up
- ❑ Salt and pepper
- ❑ Flour
- ❑ Shortening
- ❑ 10 tablespoons of flour
- ❑ 1 onion, chopped
- ❑ 3 quarts of water
- ❑ 4 stalks of celery, chopped

1. Season fryer with salt and pepper; sprinkle with flour.

2. Sauté in enough shortening to cover bottom of pot until dark golden brown; place in six-quart soup pot.

3. Drain all shortening from skillet, leaving residue at bottom; reserve drippings.

4. Add six tablespoons of the drippings and ten tablespoons of flour to skillet and brown until dark golden brown, about 10 or 15 minutes, being careful not to burn.

5. When browned, add onion and cook until limp; add this to cooked chicken, then add water and celery.

6. Bring to a boil, reduce heat to simmering and cook about two hours, stirring occasionally; season with salt and pepper.

7. Remove chicken, debone, skin and put meat back into gumbo.

8. Serve over hot rice.

– Mrs. Paul Sewall, Jr.
Lafayette (Lafayette Parish)

Fresh Vegetable Soup

- ❏ 1½ to 2 pounds of fresh beef brisket
- ❏ 4 quarts of water (to start)
- ❏ 1 tablespoon of salt
- ❏ 1 teaspoon of Tabasco
- ❏ 4 cups of onion, coarsely chopped
- ❏ 3 cups of celery, cut in 1-inch pieces
- ❏ 1 cup of tomato, peeled and cut in 1-inch pieces
- ❏ 2 cups of fresh carrots, cut in 1/2-inch pieces
- ❏ 1½ cups of bellpepper, cut in 1-inch pieces
- ❏ 1½ cups of cabbage, coarsely chopped
- ❏ 1 cup of fresh green beans, cut in 1-inch pieces
- ❏ 2 tablespoons of tomato paste
- ❏ 2 cups of green onion, coarsely chopped

1. Place the brisket, water, salt and hot pepper sauce in a six-quart stock pot and bring to a rapid boil. Boil for 30 minutes, skimming the scum that appears from time to time. Lower heat to medium.

2. Add half of the onion (two cups) and all the celery, tomato and carrot. Add enough water to bring liquid to original water line. Boil 20 minutes. Add more water, bringing liquid to original water level.

3. Add the remaining two cups of onion and all the bellpepper, cabbage, green beans and tomato paste. Boil 20 minutes. Add water, bringing liquid to original water line.

4. Add the green onion and boil for five minutes.

5. To serve, remove brisket to shallow pan. Cut into one-and-a-half-inch cubes and place in serving bowls. Ladle soup into each bowl.

Note: For a side dish of brisket, set aside desired portion and slice it into thin slices. Serve three or four slices per plate. Ladle one-fourth cup of soup over each serving. Place one teaspoon of horseradish at the edge of each plate. Serve with the soup.

– Randolph's Restaurant
Golden Meadow (Lafourche Parish)

Stuffed bellpeppers are prepared by Cajun cook Rose Broussard of Youngsville, La., which is just down the road from Lafayette.

CHICKEN & SAUSAGE JAMBALAYA

- ❑ 1 six-pound hen, cut for frying
- ❑ 1 tablespoon of salt
- ❑ ½ tablespoon of black pepper
- ❑ ½ tablespoon of red pepper
- ❑ 1 cup of oil
- ❑ 1 large onion, minced
- ❑ 3 garlic cloves, minced
- ❑ 2 pounds of smoked sausage, cut into 1-inch pieces
- ❑ 3 quarts of water
- ❑ 1 bunch of green onions, chopped
- ❑ Parsley, chopped
- ❑ 6 cups of short-grain rice, uncooked

1. Season chicken with salt and pepper.

2. In a large black iron pot, brown chicken in oil.

3. Add onions and garlic; cook until onions are clear.

4. Remove chicken, onions and garlic from pot.

5. Add sausage to oil and brown quickly.

6. Remove sausage and excess oil from pot.

7. Add chicken, onions, garlic, sausage and water to pot; cover pot and cook until chicken is tender, skimming excess fat from water. (Be sure there are at least 12 cups of stock in the pot.)

8. Add onion tops, parsley and rice; bring to rapid boil, stir and taste for seasoning.

9. Lower heat, cover and cook for 30 to 45 minutes or until rice is cooked and stock absorbed.

– Mrs. Sandy Hebert
Lafayette (Lafayette Parish)

PORK FRICASSEE

- ❑ Water
- ❑ 5 tablespoons of roux
- ❑ 3 large onions, chopped
- ❑ 3 pounds of pork steak
- ❑ Salt and pepper
- ❑ 1 bunch of green onions, chopped

1. Add enough water to roux to make a thick gravy in skillet; add onion and pork, then season, to taste.

2. Simmer until tender; add green onions and serve over rice.

– Manning "Pete" Broussard
Lafayette (Lafayette Parish)

ℭHICKEN STEW

- ❏ 2 tablespoons of butter
- ❏ ½ cup of flour
- ❏ 1 onion, chopped
- ❏ 1 bellpepper, chopped
- ❏ 1 rib of celery, chopped
- ❏ ½ cup of chopped parsley
- ❏ 2 cups of water
- ❏ 1 chicken, cut up
- ❏ Salt and pepper, to taste
- ❏ 1 teaspoon of garlic salt

1. Make a roux with butter and flour in pot; add onion, bellpepper, celery and parsley; cook until wilted.

2. Add water, chicken and seasonings; cook about 25 minutes or until chicken is done.

Serve over rice.

– Mrs. Mary Colar
Franklin (St. Mary Parish)

*R*ED BEANS AND RICE

- ❑ 1 pound of red beans, sorted and washed
- ❑ ¾ pound of pickled pork, sliced
- ❑ 1 medium onion, chopped
- ❑ ¼ bellepepper, chopped
- ❑ Salt and pepper, to taste
- ❑ Cooked rice

1. Soak beans overnight in water to cover.

2. In same soaking water, bring beans to a boil; lower heat and simmer for one and one-half to two hours.

3. Add pickled pork, onion, bellpepper and salt and pepper, to taste; simmer another hour and a half or until beans and pork are tender.

4. Serve over cooked rice.

– Myrtle McDonough
New Iberia (Iberia Parish)

SAUSAGE JAMBALAYA

- ❏ 2 pounds of smoked sausage
- ❏ ½ cup of oil
- ❏ 1 large onion, chopped
- ❏ 2 stalks of celery, chopped
- ❏ 1 medium bellpepper, chopped
- ❏ 2 cups of uncooked rice
- ❏ 4 cups of water
- ❏ Salt, black pepper and cayenne, to taste
- ❏ Green onions and parsley, to taste

1. Cut smoked sausage into four-inch links and boil in two quarts of water for 25 minutes. Pour out excess water and slice sausage into bite-size pieces.

2. Brown sausage in heavy skillet in cooking oil until well-browned.

3. Add onion, celery and bellpepper and cook until onion is transparent.

4. Add rice and water, along with seasonings. Cover and cook over low heat, stirring frequently. (If rice does not seem to be cooking thoroughly through the process, continue adding water in small amounts until cooked and no longer mushy, perhaps one hour.)

5. Add green onions and parsley just before serving.

– Mrs. Donald J. Dooley
Jeanerette (Iberia Parish)

CHICKEN FRICASSEE

- ❑ 1 tablespoon of margarine
- ❑ 1 large onion, chopped
- ❑ 1 medium bellpepper, chopped
- ❑ 3 cloves of garlic, chopped
- ❑ 3 cups of chicken stock or canned chicken broth
- ❑ ½ cup of dry roux mixed with 1 cup of water to form a paste
- ❑ 1 large fryer, cut up and skinned
- ❑ Salt, black pepper, and red pepper, to taste
- ❑ ½ cup of onion tops, chopped
- ❑ ¼ cup of parsley, chopped

1. Heat heavy-bottom pot on medium heat. Add margarine, onion, bellpepper and garlic. Cook until soft.

2. Add chicken stock or broth. Bring to a boil. Add roux mixture. Cook about 20 minutes.

3. Add chicken pieces and seasonings. Cook about 30 minutes.

4. Add onion tops and parsley. Cook 10 minutes more.

5. Serve over rice.

– Carol Vincent
Lafayette (Lafayette Parish)

STUFFED MIRLITON

- ❏ 5 medium-size mirlitons (vegetable pears)
- ❏ ¼ cup of grated fresh onion
- ❏ ¾ cup of finely chopped green onion tops
- ❏ 3 garlic cloves, minced
- ❏ ¼ cup of snipped parsley
- ❏ ½ cup of bacon grease
- ❏ ½ cup of ground cooked ham
- ❏ ½ cup of raw shrimp, chopped fine
- ❏ 1 cup of cooked rice
- ❏ ½ teaspoon of salt
- ❏ ¼ teaspoon of cayenne pepper
- ❏ 1 teaspoon of monosodium glutamate
- ❏ 1 egg, beaten
- ❏ Buttered breadcrumbs

1. Cover mirlitons with water, boil until tender (about one hour). Cool; cut in half length-wise. Scoop out pulp and reserve. Discard seeds and set shells aside for stuffing.

2. Sauté onions, green onions, garlic and parsley in bacon grease. Add ham and shrimp; cook, stirring gently for five minutes.

3. Add mirliton pulp, rice and seasonings. Cook 10 minutes. Add more bacon grease if too dry. Remove from heat.

4. Add egg; return to heat; cook one minute.

5. Fill shells, sprinkle with buttered fresh breadcrumbs.

6. Bake uncovered at 375 degrees for 15 to 20 minutes or until crumbs are browned.

Serves five.

– Mrs. Youngs Foreman
Indian Bayou (Vermilion Parish)

Tourtiere
(Pork Pie)

- ❑ 2 pounds of ground lean pork
- ❑ ½ cup of chopped onion
- ❑ 1 cup of chopped celery
- ❑ 1 garlic clove, crushed
- ❑ ¼ cup of chopped parsley
- ❑ 1 teaspoon of salt
- ❑ ¼ teaspoon of leaf marjoram, crushed
- ❑ ¼ teaspoon of ground cloves
- ❑ ¼ teaspoon of ground mace
- ❑ ½ teaspoon of ground pepper
- ❑ 2 tablespoons of flour
- ❑ 2 beef bouillon cubes
- ❑ 1 cup of hot water
- ❑ Pastry for 2-crust pie, unbaked
  (can use frozen pie shells)

1. Sauté pork, onion, celery and garlic in a large skillet until pork is brown and vegetables are tender.

2. Stir in parsley, salt, marjoram, cloves, mace and pepper; cover and simmer over low heat for 30 minutes.

3. Drain excess fat from skillet; blend flour into meat mixture. Add bouillon cubes dissolved in hot water.

4. Return to heat and bring mixture to a boil; simmer for one minute, stirring constantly. Remove from heat and set aside to cool.

5. Pile meat mixture in pie shell; top with other shell, seal and flute edges. (Brush with egg if desired.)

6. Bake at 400 degrees for 45 minutes or until golden brown.

Makes one nine-inch pie.

Serves six.

Can be eaten warm or cold.

– Mrs. Hazel Gourgues
Hahnville (St. Charles Parish)

GRILLADES

- ❑ 1 garlic clove, mashed
- ❑ 1 tablespoon of oil
- ❑ 2 quarts of green onion tops, chopped
- ❑ 1 4- to 5-pound pork roast, cut into pieces
  ½-inch thick by 3 inches square
- ❑ 1 large onion, chopped
- ❑ Salt and pepper, to taste

1. Spread garlic on the sides and bottom of a large bowl. Pour oil in the bowl.

2. Place in layers the green onions and then about two inches of meat. Continue layers, using all the green onions and all the meat, ending with the green onions.

3. Cover tightly and keep in the refrigerator for a day or two.

4. Take out amount desired and place in a large pot with a small amount of oil. Add onions and some of the green onion tops. Season to taste. Let brown, adding water as needed. Cook on low heat until tender.

– Mrs. Jessie Hoffpauir
Indian Bayou (Vermilion Parish)

*S*TUFFED *B*ELLPEPPERS

- ½ pound of ground meat (or shrimp, pork or veal may be used)
- 2 tablespoons of fat
- 1 onion, chopped
- 2 tablespoons of chopped bellpepper
- ½ cup of canned tomato (or 1 fresh tomato), peeled and chopped
- 1 cup of water
- 1 cup of cooked rice (or breadcrumbs)
- Salt and pepper, to taste
- 6 whole bellpeppers
- ½ cup of buttered breadcrumbs

1. Brown meat in fat; add onion and chopped bellpepper. Cook until onions are tender.

2. Add tomato and water; cook until meat is tender. Add rice or breadcrumbs and seasonings, to taste.

3. Cut off stem ends of whole bellpeppers and remove seeds; boil bellpeppers for five minutes in lightly salted water; drain.

4. Stuff bellpepper with meat mixture; cover with buttered breadcrumbs.

5. Bake at 350 degrees for 20 minutes.

– Mrs. Francis Kerne
Thibodaux (Lafourche Parish)

*L*IVER AND ONIONS

- ❑ 2 pounds of calf liver
- ❑ 2 teaspoons of baking soda
- ❑ 2 cups of boiling water
- ❑ 1 teaspoon of salt
- ❑ ½ teaspoon of pepper
- ❑ ½ cup of flour
- ❑ ½ cup of oil
- ❑ 2 onions, chopped
- ❑ 1 teaspoon of hot pepper sauce

1. Place liver in large flat pan; sprinkle with soda. Pour rapidly boiling water over liver; stir until well-mixed.

2. Pour off hot water; rinse liver well with cold water.

3. Sprinkle salt and pepper on liver; roll in flour.

4. Brown liver quickly in hot oil; remove liver from skillet and pour out oil.

5. Return liver to skillet, alternating with layers of onion. Sprinkle with pepper sauce; add enough water to make a gravy, one to two cups.

6. Cover and cook on low heat 15 to 20 minutes, stirring once or twice to prevent sticking.

– June Crain Harper
Grand Chenier (Cameron Parish)

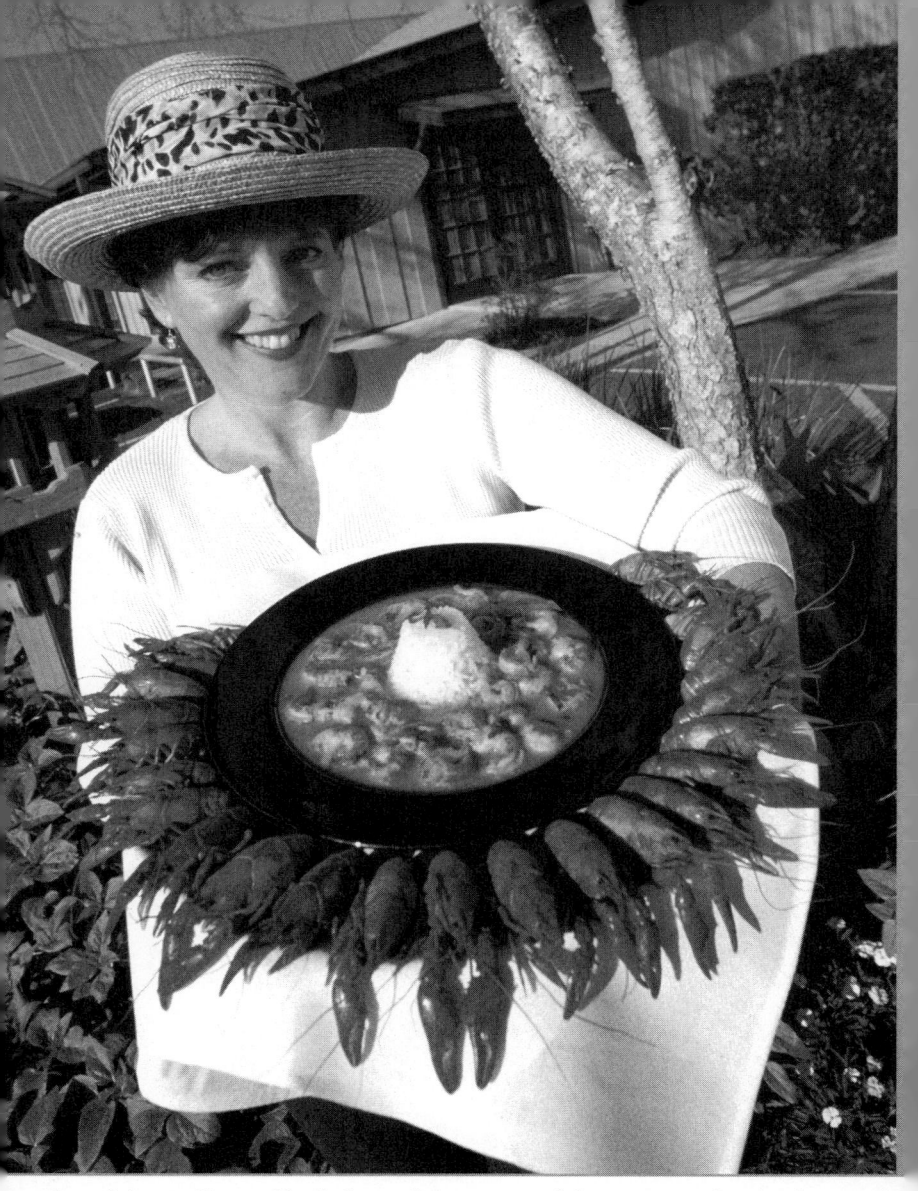

Crawfish etouffee and boiled crawfish are two of the most popular foods served in the Cajun country of south Louisiana.

CRAWFISH PIE

- ☐ ¾ medium bellpepper, chopped
- ☐ 1 large onion, chopped
- ☐ 2 ribs of celery, chopped
- ☐ ¾ cup of butter
- ☐ 6 tablespoons of crawfish fat (optional)
- ☐ 1½ pounds of peeled crawfish tails
- ☐ ½ cup of chopped green onions
- ☐ ½ cup of minced parsley
- ☐ 1½ teaspoons of salt
- ☐ ½ teaspoon of black pepper
- ☐ ¼ teaspoon of red pepper
- ☐ ½ teaspoon of garlic powder
- ☐ Cornstarch
- ☐ Dough for a double-crust pie

1. Sauté bellpepper, onion and celery in butter until tender; add crawfish fat and simmer 10 minutes.

2. Add crawfish tails, green onions, parsley and seasonings. Thicken if necessary with a little cornstarch; let cook long enough to thicken gravy.

3. Place half of the pie crust dough in a nine-inch pie pan. Fill with the cooled filling. Place top crust on pie, moisten edges and seal edges. Cut two or three one-inch-long slits in the top crust.

4. Bake 10 minutes at 450 degrees; lower oven to 375 degrees and cook for 35 minutes longer or until crust is golden brown.

Note: Individual pies can be made using muffin pans with large cups. Bake as above.

– LSU Cooperative Extension Service
Iberville Parish

CRABMEAT AU GRATIN

- ❑ ½ cup of chopped green onions
- ❑ 2 tablespoons of chopped celery
- ❑ ½ cup of chopped mushrooms
- ❑ 3 tablespoons of butter
- ❑ 1 cup of thick White Sauce (Recipe follows)
- ❑ 1 pound of lump crabmeat
- ❑ Salt and Tabasco sauce, to taste
- ❑ 1 cup of American cheese, grated

1. Sauté chopped green onions, celery and mushrooms in butter.

2. Add White Sauce, crabmeat, salt and Tabasco.

3. Place in buttered baking dish, top with cheese and bake at 350 degrees until brown, about 20 to 25 minutes.

4. Garnish with black olive halves and wedges of lemon.

WHITE SAUCE

- ❑ ¼ cup of butter
- ❑ ¼ cup of flour
- ❑ 1 cup of milk, scalded
- ❑ Salt and pepper, to taste

1. Melt butter in heavy saucepan; blend-in flour on low heat, stirring constantly until smooth.

2. Remove from heat; stir-in heated milk a little at a time.

3. Season, to taste; cook on low heat until thick and bubbly.

– Mrs. Martha Montrejean
Cut Off (Lafourche Parish)

SHRIMP SALAD

- ❑ ¾ cup of mayonnaise
- ❑ 1 teaspoon of salt
- ❑ 2 teaspoons of dry mustard
- ❑ 6 green onions, minced or diced
- ❑ 2 stalks of celery, minced
- ❑ 1 teaspoon of paprika
- ❑ 2 drops of hot sauce
- ❑ 3 sprigs of parsley, minced
- ❑ 2 pounds of shrimp, boiled and peeled
- ❑ Lettuce leaves
- ❑ Hard-boiled eggs, halved

1. Combine first eight ingredients and pour over shrimp; refrigerate for four to six hours.

2. Serve on lettuce leaves and decorate with eggs.

– Agnes Mahen
Hahnville (St. Charles Parish)

$\mathcal{S}$TEAMED SHRIMP

- ❑ ¼ cup of red wine vinegar
- ❑ ½ cup of olive oil
- ❑ 4 green onions, chopped
- ❑ 1 large onion, chopped
- ❑ ½ rib of celery, chopped
- ❑ 2 lemons, sliced thick
- ❑ Salt, pepper and garlic powder, to taste
- ❑ 4 pounds of raw shrimp,
  unpeeled but de-headed

1. Mix all ingredients together in large pot; stir well.

2. Cover and simmer about 45 minutes; stir often.

– Mrs. Gordon Martin
Grand Point (St. James Parish)

*B*OILED SHRIMP

- ❑ 1 gallon of water
- ❑ 1 lemon, sliced thin
- ❑ 1 onion, sliced
- ❑ ¼ cup of cayenne pepper
- ❑ 3 pounds of shrimp (leave peelings on)
- ❑ 1 cup of salt

1. Bring water, lemons, onion and cayenne pepper to a boil in a large pot; simmer for five to ten minutes.

2. Add shrimp; bring to a boil for three minutes only.

3. Remove from heat and add one cup of cold water (to stop the boiling process) and salt to pot of shrimp; let stand for five minutes and drain.

Makes four to six servings.

*B*AKED *SHRIMP*

- ❏ 5 pounds of shrimp, unpeeled and heads on (medium preferred)
- ❏ 3 tablespoons of salt
- ❏ 6 lemons, sliced
- ❏ ¼ pound of butter, melted
- ❏ Pepper sauce and paprika, to taste

1. Wash shrimp well; arrange in shallow pan, 12 x 6 x 2.

2. Add remaining ingredients.

3. Cover with foil and bake at 350 degrees for 45 minutes.

4. About 20 minutes before shrimp are done, remove foil, stir and continue to bake with foil off the pan. Taste shrimp for doneness, as sometimes larger shrimp require longer baking.

5. The juice is served in a small bowl to each guest for dunking hot, buttered French bread.

– Georgiana Bourg
Donaldsonville (Ascension Parish)

*B*ROILED *S*HRIMP

- ❑ 1 pound of raw shrimp, peeled
- ❑ Salt and pepper, to taste
- ❑ ¼ cup of butter
- ❑ Juice of one lemon
- ❑ Worcestershire sauce (optional)
- ❑ Parsley, chopped

1. Place seasoned shrimp in shallow pan; dot butter on top of shrimp and squeeze on juice of one-half lemon.

2. Place in broiler about four inches from heat source; broil for three minutes.

3. Turn each shrimp over. (If Worcestershire sauce will be used, sprinkle on shrimp about two minutes before turning.)

4. After turning, squeeze juice of remainder of lemon on shrimp.

5. Broil about seven minutes or until brown.

6. Sprinkle parsley on shrimp after removing from heat.

Serve immediately.

– Mrs. Cleo Cheramie
Golden Meadow (Lafourche Parish)

*F*RIED SHRIMP

- ☐ 1 cup of flour
- ☐ Salt and pepper, to taste
- ☐ 2 eggs
- ☐ ¼ cup of milk
- ☐ 2 teaspoons of mustard, preferably with onion bits
- ☐ 3 or 4 pounds of peeled shrimp
- ☐ Vegetable oil

1. Season the flour heavily with salt and pepper.

2. Beat eggs and milk together; add mustard; season mixture with salt and pepper; add a little flour to thicken.

3. Dip shrimp in egg mixture then roll in flour.

4. Over medium heat in one-half inch of oil, fry shrimp for two or three minutes on each side until golden brown, being careful not to overcook.

5. Drain on paper towels or brown paper bag.

Serves six.

– Sidney Richard
Franklin (St. Mary Parish)

$\mathcal{S}$HRIMP STEW

- ❑ 1 onion, chopped
- ❑ ½ cup of chopped bellpepper
- ❑ ½ cup of chopped celery
- ❑ 4 tablespoons of oil
- ❑ 1¾ pounds of peeled shrimp
- ❑ 3½ cups of water
- ❑ 3 tablespoons of flour
- ❑ 1 tablespoon of liquid brown gravy coloring
  (like Kitchen Bouquet)
- ❑ Salt and pepper, to taste

1. Sauté onions, bellpeppers and celery in oil; add shrimp and simmer five minutes on a low heat.

2. Add three cups of the water and bring to a boil.

3. Mix flour and one-half cup of the water until it is smooth; add to the shrimp mixture.

4. Reduce heat and continue stirring until thoroughly mixed; add liquid brown gravy coloring and simmer 15 minutes.

5. Serve over hot rice.

Serves six.

– Mollie Prince
Ascension Parish

*S*TUFFED *S*HRIMP

- ❑ 1 cup of oil
- ❑ 1 cup of chopped onion
- ❑ 1 cup of chopped bellpepper
- ❑ 1 cup of chopped celery
- ❑ 1 pound of crabmeat
- ❑ Salt and pepper, to taste
- ❑ Breadcrumbs
- ❑ 1 pound of large shrimp, peeled (leave on tips of tails and last segment of shells)
- ❑ 2 eggs
- ❑ 1 cup of evaporated milk
- ❑ Corn flour
- ❑ Oil of frying

1. Sauté in oil the onion, bellpepper and celery until tender.

2. Add crabmeat, seasonings, a small amount of water and breadcrumbs to make a stiff dressing.

3. "Butterfly" the shrimp by making a vertical cut in the back; stuff center with dressing, squeezing shrimp in hand to form a croquette. Freeze shrimp.

4. Mix eggs and evaporated milk; dip frozen shrimp into egg-milk mixture, then into corn flour.

5. Fry while frozen in deep oil until brown.

Note: Crabs and flounder can be stuffed with the same dressing.

– Mrs. Amelie Naquin
New Iberia (Iberia Parish)

SHRIMP & OYSTERS EN BROCHETTE

- ¼ pound of butter
- 2 cloves of garlic, minced
- 1 lemon
- 1 pound of large shrimp, peeled and deveined
- Salt and cayenne, to taste
- ½ slice of bacon for each shrimp
- 3 dozen oysters

1. Melt butter and add garlic and the juice of the lemon. Heat to boiling and stir. Reduce heat.

2. Split shrimp, if desired. Season each individually with salt and cayenne.

3. Wrap each shrimp with half a slice of bacon and secure with toothpick.

4. Alternate shrimp with oysters on six skewers.

5. Place skewers in shallow pan about five inches from flame of broiling oven and broil 15 to 20 minutes, until bacon is crisp.

6. Baste with butter sauce and turn frequently.

7. Serve with tartar sauce.

Serves six.

– Don's Seafood & Steak House
Lafayette (Lafayette Parish)

*F*RIED OYSTERS

- ❑ 1 egg, beaten
- ❑ 3 tablespoons of baking powder
- ❑ Cayenne pepper, to taste
- ❑ 2 pints of fresh oysters, drained
- ❑ 1½ cups of flour
- ❑ ¼ cup of chopped parsley
- ❑ Oil for frying

1. Combine egg, baking powder and cayenne pepper and mix well; soak oysters in this mixture.

2. Combine flour, parsley and cayenne pepper; dip oysters in this mixture and shake off excess flour.

3. Fry in deep, hot oil at 375 degrees until golden brown; drain on paper towels.

Makes four to six servings.

${\mathcal B}$OILED CRAWFISH

- ❑ 20 pounds of live crawfish
- ❑ ½ box of salt
- ❑ 6 lemons, cut in wedges
- ❑ 3 pounds of onions, cut in wedges
- ❑ 1½ boxes of salt
- ❑ ¼ bottle of liquid crab boil
- ❑ ¼ bottle of red pepper

1. Place live crawfish into a large tub. Add one-half box of salt and enough water to cover them. Leave crawfish in tub for 20 to 30 minutes, to allow them to rinse and purge.

2. Fill a large seafood-boiling pot about one-third full of water; add all remaining ingredients except crawfish and bring water to a brisk boil for about 10 minutes.

3. Pour the crawfish into the pot. After the water comes to a boil again, let it boil for about seven minutes.

4. Cut off the fire and let the crawfish soak for five or 10 minutes before serving.

CRAWFISH FETTUCCINE

- ❑ 1 stick of butter
- ❑ 1 cup of chopped onion
- ❑ 1 cup of chopped bellpepper
- ❑ 3 pounds of crawfish tails
- ❑ 1 pint of crawfish fat
- ❑ 2 tablespoons of salt
- ❑ 1 teaspoon of white pepper
- ❑ 1 tablespoon of red pepper
- ❑ 1 tablespoon of seafood seasoning
- ❑ Chopped parsley
- ❑ 1½ pounds of fettuccine noodles

1. Melt butter in heavy pot. Add onion and bellpepper; sauté till tender.

2. Add crawfish tails and cook about 10 minutes.

3. Add fat, salt, pepper and seafood seasoning, and cook two or three minutes more. Add parsley.

4. Boil the fettuccine noodles according to package directions; drain and place in a bowl.

5. Add cooked crawfish and desired amount of Sauce (Recipe follows). Toss lightly.

6. Place in casserole, top with breadcrumbs and bake uncovered at 350 for 10 minutes or until breadcrumbs are brown.

- ❑ 4 cups of evaporated milk
- ❑ 1 tablespoon of garlic powder
- ❑ 1 tablespoon of nutmeg
- ❑ 2 cups of Parmesan cheese
- ❑ Chopped parsley

1. Place evaporated milk in heavy pot and bring to a boil.

2. Add garlic powder, nutmeg, cheese and parsley.

3. Remove from stove to cool. It thickens as it cools.

Serves eight to ten.

– Forest Restaurant
Franklin (St. Mary Parish)

CRAWFISH ETOUFFEE

- ❑ 1 cup of chopped green onions
- ❑ 1 cup of chopped celery
- ❑ ¼ pound of oleo
- ❑ 3 tablespoons of flour
- ❑ Crawfish fat
- ❑ 1 can of chicken broth
- ❑ 1 pound of crawfish tails
- ❑ Salt, black pepper and red pepper, to taste
- ❑ 2 teaspoons of paprika
- ❑ Green onion tops, chopped
- ❑ Parsley, chopped

1. Sauté onions and celery in oleo until wilted. Add flour and cook, but do not brown.

2. Add crawfish fat and chicken broth; simmer 20 minutes.

3. Add crawfish tails, salt, pepper and paprika; simmer 20 minutes more.

4. Before serving, add onion tops and parsley.

– Jeanette M. Guidry
Breaux Bridge (St. Martin Parish)

FRIED CATFISH

- 1½ cups of yellow cornmeal
- 2½ cups of flour
- ½ cup of chopped parsley
- Salt and cayenne pepper, to taste
- 2 pounds of catfish filets
- Oil for frying

1. Combine cornmeal, flour, parsley, salt and cayenne pepper.

2. Season catfish and dip into cornmeal mixture, shaking off excess flour.

3. Fry in hot, deep oil at 375 degrees until golden brown; drain on paper towels.

Makes four to six servings.

*B*AKED STUFFED CATFISH

- ❑ 2 onions, chopped
- ❑ 4 stalks of celery, chopped
- ❑ 1 bellpepper, chopped
- ❑ ½ cup of butter
- ❑ 2 10-ounce cans of tomatoes with chilies
- ❑ 1 8-ounce can of tomato sauce
- ❑ Salt, black pepper and cayenne pepper, to taste
- ❑ ¼ cup of chopped parsley
- ❑ ¼ cup of chopped green onion tops
- ❑ 1 5-pound whole catfish,
  cleaned and head removed
- ❑ Shrimp and Crab Stuffing (Recipe follows)

1. Sauté onion, celery and bellpepper in butter until onions are transparent; add remaining ingredients except fish and stuffing and simmer about 20 to 30 minutes.

2. Season fish with salt, black pepper and cayenne pepper and stuff cavity with Shrimp and Crab Stuffing.

3. Place stuffed fish in a foil-lined baking dish and pour tomato mixture over the top; close foil over fish tightly and bake at 350 degrees for about 30 to 45 minutes.

Makes four to six servings.

SHRIMP AND CRAB STUFFING

- ❑ 1 onion, chopped
- ❑ ½ bellpepper, chopped
- ❑ ¼ cup of oil
- ❑ ½ pound of peeled and deveined shrimp
- ❑ ½ pound of crabmeat
- ❑ Salt, black pepper and cayenne pepper, to taste
- ❑ ¼ cup of water

1. Sauté onion and bellpepper in oil until onions are transparent.

2. Add shrimp, crabmeat, salt, black pepper, cayenne pepper and water and simmer five minutes.

$\mathcal{L}$OUISIANA SEAFOOD SAUCE PIQUANTE

- ❑ 1½ cups of vegetable oil
- ❑ 2 cups of all-purpose flour
- ❑ 2 cups of chopped onion
- ❑ 2 garlic cloves, minced
- ❑ ½ cup of chopped green bellpepper
- ❑ ¼ cup of chopped celery
- ❑ 2 pounds of catfish fillets
- ❑ 1 can (8 ounces) of Rotel tomatoes with chilies, diced
- ❑ 1 can (4 ounces) of tomato sauce
- ❑ 1 can (10¾ ounces) of cream of mushroom soup
- ❑ 2 quarts of water
- ❑ 1 pound of peeled raw shrimp
- ❑ 1 pound of lump crabmeat
- ❑ 1 tablespoon of seasoned salt
- ❑ ½ teaspoon of salt
- ❑ ½ teaspoon of black pepper
- ❑ 1 cup of chopped green onion
- ❑ ¼ cup of parsley

1. In a heavy sauce pot (10 quarts) make a roux by combining oil and flour over medium heat, stirring constantly until golden brown.

2. Add onion, garlic, green bellpepper, and celery to roux and continue cooking for about 15 minutes.

3. Cut one pound of catfish into small pieces and add to roux.

4. After about five minutes, add Rotel tomatoes, tomato sauce, cream of mushroom soup, and water.

5. Allow to simmer for about one hour, stirring often to avoid sticking.

6. While sauce is simmering, bake remaining one pound of catfish on sheet pan for 20 minutes at 400 degrees. (This will firm up the catfish.)

7. At the end of the one hour of simmering, add shrimp, catfish (baked) and lump crabmeat.

8. Continue cooking for approximately 20 minutes or until catfish, shrimp, and crab are done.

9. Add seasoned salt, salt and pepper.

10. Green onion and parsley should be added about 15 minutes before sauce piquante is done.

11. Serve over rice.

Makes 18 servings.

– Jerry Folse
Donaldsonville (Ascension Parish)

CATFISH SAUCE PIQUANTE

- ❑ 4 to 5 pounds of fish
- ❑ 2 cups of chopped onions
- ❑ ½ cup of oil
- ❑ 1 cup of chopped celery
- ❑ 2 garlic cloves, minced
- ❑ 1 bellpepper, chopped
- ❑ 1 can of tomato paste
- ❑ 1 can of tomato sauce
- ❑ Juice and rind of 1 lemon
- ❑ 1 teaspoon of salt
- ❑ Cayenne pepper, to taste
- ❑ ¼ cup of green onions, chopped
- ❑ ¼ cup of parsley, chopped

1. Boil fish long enough to debone easily; save fish stock for later use.

2. Sauté onions in oil until transparent; add celery, garlic, bellpepper, tomato paste, tomato sauce, lemon rind, salt and cayenne pepper.

3. Cook 45 minutes on low heat.

4. Add one cup of fish stock or more if it is too thick.

5. Add lemon juice, green onions and parsley.

6. Add fish to sauce and simmer for 15 to 20 minutes.

7. Serve over rice.

Serves six to eight.

– Tess Cavell
Ventress (Pointe Coupee Parish)

CRABMEAT IMPERIAL

- ❑ ½ pound of butter or oleo
- ❑ 1 cup of flour
- ❑ 2 cups of milk
- ❑ ½ cup of celery, chopped fine
- ❑ ½ cup of mushrooms, chopped fine
- ❑ ½ cup of parsley, chopped fine
- ❑ ½ cup of green onions, chopped fine
- ❑ ½ cup of pimientos, chopped fine
- ❑ 2 pounds of lump crabmeat
- ❑ Worcestershire sauce, to taste
- ❑ Tabasco sauce, to taste
- ❑ Salt and pepper, to taste
- ❑ Breadcrumbs

1. Melt butter over low heat and stir-in flour. Cook until bubbles appear on top.

2. Add milk slowly, stirring constantly.

3. Add celery and mushrooms.

4. Continue cooking while adding parsley, green onions and pimientos.

5. Fold-in crabmeat.

6. Add Worcestershire sauce, hot pepper sauce, salt and pepper, to taste.

7. Pour mixture into individual baking dishes and sprinkle with breadcrumbs.

8. Bake until brown in 350-degree oven.

– Riverside Inn
Broussard (Lafayette Parish)

*S*TUFFED *C*RABS

- ❑ 1 cup of chopped onions
- ❑ ½ cup of chopped celery
- ❑ ½ cup of chopped bellpepper
- ❑ 2 garlic cloves, minced
- ❑ ¼ pound of oleo or ½ cup of oil
- ❑ ½ teaspoon of Worcestershire sauce
- ❑ 1 pound of crabmeat (about 10 crabs)
- ❑ Salt, black pepper and red pepper, to taste
- ❑ ½ cup of chopped green onion tops
- ❑ 1 tablespoon of chopped parsley
- ❑ 2 stale hamburger buns
  (or 6 slices of stale bread)
- ❑ 1 cup of evaporated milk
- ❑ 3 eggs
- ❑ Breadcrumbs

1. Sauté onion, celery, bellpepper and garlic in oleo or oil until wilted.

2. Add Worcestershire sauce, crabmeat and seasoning, to taste; cook over medium heat about 15 minutes, stirring constantly.

3. Add onion tops, parsley and bread which has been soaked in milk-and-egg mixture; mix well.

4. Fill 12 crab shells; top with breadcrumbs.

5. Bake 15 minutes at 375 degrees.

– Mary Campbell
Ascension Parish

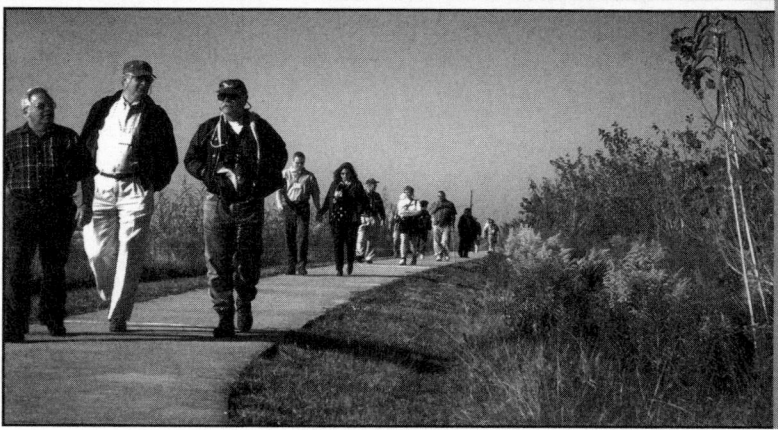

The Creole Nature Trail in the southwest corner of Louisiana is an All-American Road featuring beautiful scenery and every manner of feathered and furry wildlife. A stroll along the Wetland Walkway provides an especially close-up look.

RABBIT IN TOMATO GRAVY

- ❑ 1 large rabbit, cut into serving pieces
- ❑ Cooking oil
- ❑ 2 onions, chopped
- ❑ 3 to 4 garlic cloves, minced
- ❑ 1 large can of tomatoes
- ❑ ½ can of tomato paste
- ❑ Parsley and green onions, chopped
- ❑ 1 can of sliced mushrooms
- ❑ Salt and pepper, to taste

1. Fry rabbit in a small amount of oil until brown; remove from pan.

2. Sauté onions and garlic with tomatoes and tomato paste; add about a cup of water when the mixture starts to stick.

3. Cook until thick, about an hour and a half.

4. Add rabbit and cook until rabbit is tender, an hour to an hour and a half; add parsley, green onions and mushrooms. Season to taste.

– Mrs. Carmen Brady
Hahnville (St. Charles Parish)

SMOTHERED FROG LEGS

- ❑ 6 pair of frog legs
- ❑ 2 tablespoons of butter
- ❑ Salt and pepper, to taste
- ❑ 4 onions, sliced
- ❑ 6 whole tomatoes, fresh or canned
- ❑ 1 bay leaf
- ❑ 1 sprig of thyme
- ❑ ¼ cup of chopped parsley
- ❑ 2 garlic cloves, pressed
- ❑ 4 bellpeppers, diced
- ❑ 1 cup of water or stock

1. Slowly brown frog legs in butter; add salt, pepper and onions and cook until brown.

2. Add tomatoes, bay leaf, thyme, parsley and garlic; cover and cook slowly for 30 minutes.

3. Add bellpeppers and water or stock; continue to smother until frog legs are tender, 45 minutes to an hour.

– Mrs. John Prescott
Johnson Bayou (Cameron Parish)

*B*aked *W*ild *D*ucks

- ❑ 2 ducks
- ❑ Salt and pepper
- ❑ 2 medium onions
- ❑ 1 celery stalk
- ❑ ¼ cup of oil
- ❑ 1 cup of water
- ❑ 1 cup of sherry
- ❑ 1 tablespoon of flour
- ❑ ¼ cup of water
- ❑ 3 tablespoons of chopped parsley

1. Season ducks with salt and pepper inside and out; stuff cavity of each duck with one-half of an onion and one-half of a stalk of celery.

2. Brown in an open heavy roasting pan at 400 degrees in oil; add remaining onion, chopped, to pan and wilt.

3. Add one cup of water and sherry; reduce heat to 350 degrees, cover and cook until tender, about two hours or more, depending on size.

4. Baste and add more liquid if needed; make a paste with flour and one-fourth cup of water and add to the drippings to make gravy. Add parsley.

– Louis "Billy" Fontenot
Jennings (Jefferson Davis Parish)

VENISON STEW

- ❑ 2 pounds of boneless venison stew meat
- ❑ Cooking oil
- ❑ Salt, pepper, and garlic powder, to taste
- ❑ 2 cans of golden mushroom soup
- ❑ 1 soup can of burgundy wine
- ❑ 1 cup of chopped bellpepper
- ❑ ½ cup of chopped celery
- ❑ ¼ cup of parsley
- ❑ 1 cup of chopped onion
- ❑ 2 packages of frozen stew vegetables
  (or fresh whole onions, carrots, and small potatoes)

1. Brown stew meat in black iron pot in a small amount of oil.

2. Add seasonings, soup, wine and vegetables.

3. Cover and bake at 200 degrees for no less than eight hours.

– Mrs. Clifford Keowen
Church Point (Acadia Parish)

ALLIGATOR SAUCE PIQUANTE

- ❑ ½ cup of flour
- ❑ 1 cup of cooking oil
- ❑ 1 large onion, chopped
- ❑ 1 garlic clove, chopped
- ❑ ½ bellpepper, chopped
- ❑ 1 large can of tomatoes
- ❑ 1 can of tomato sauce
- ❑ 3 cups of water
- ❑ 1 pound of alligator, cut into one-inch cubes
- ❑ Salt and pepper, to taste
- ❑ ½ cup of onion tops, chopped

1. Cook flour in oil until medium brown; add onion and cook until onion wilts.

2. Add garlic, bellpepper, tomatoes, tomato sauce and water. Cook over low heat for 30 minutes.

3. Add meat, salt and pepper, and onion tops; continue cooking until meat is tender, about 30 to 45 minutes.

– John Prescott
Johnson Bayou (Cameron Parish)

*R*OASTED *S*QUIRREL

- ❑ ½ pound of smoked bacon, cubed
- ❑ 4 squirrels, cut in pieces
- ❑ 2 medium onions, chopped
- ❑ 1 stalk of celery, chopped
- ❑ 4 cups of chicken broth
- ❑ Salt, to taste
- ❑ Pinch of thyme
- ❑ Dash or two of hot pepper sauce

1. Brown bacon; remove and set aside.

2. Brown squirrel in drippings left from browning bacon; remove and set aside.

3. Add onions and celery to drippings and sauté two minutes.

4. Add squirrel and bacon and enough chicken broth to cover bottom of pot; add seasonings.

5. Cover and cook on a low heat, adding broth a little at a time as it needs replacing until squirrel is tender, about an hour.

Serves four.

Note: This is an ideal way to cook older squirrels that are tough. Rabbit may be cooked in this manner also.

– Mrs. Charles F. Hebert
Cameron (Cameron Parish)

Oak Alley

San Francisco

Houmas House

Nottoway

Destrehan

A number of mansions reminiscent of the antebellum South can be seen along the River Road between Baton Rouge and New Orleans. These five and others are open for tours.

Shrimp & Eggplant Dressing or Casserole

- ❑ 2 to 3 eggplants
- ❑ Hot water
- ❑ Salt
- ❑ 1 cup of water
- ❑ Red pepper and black pepper
- ❑ 1 pound of peeled shrimp, cut up
- ❑ Oleo
- ❑ 1 medium onion, chopped
- ❑ ½ cup of chopped celery
- ❑ 1 medium bellpepper, chopped
- ❑ 5 cups of cooked rice
- ❑ Breadcrumbs

1. Peel and cut up eggplants (throw away seeds if large); put in hot water with a little salt and soak for 30 minutes. Throw away this water.

2. Put eggplant in pot with one cup of water and cook down, leaving some liquid to help moisten dressing; set aside.

3. Season shrimp; sauté in a small amount of oleo until shrimp turn pink, about 10 minutes, and set aside.

4. Sauté onion, celery, and bellpepper in more oleo and add to shrimp; combine shrimp mixture, eggplant and rice, mixing well.

5. Pour into a buttered baking dish; sprinkle top with breadcrumbs.

6. Bake uncovered for 25 to 30 minutes at 350 degrees.

Note: Great for stuffing bellpeppers and tomato shells. Sautéed seasoned ground beef can be substituted for shrimp.

– Ellis Cormier
Jennings (Jefferson Davis Parish)

$\mathcal{L}$OUISIANA CORNBREAD DRESSING

- ❏ Giblets (gizzard, liver and heart)
- ❏ 2 cups of celery, cut fine
- ❏ 1½ cups of shallots with tops, cut fine
- ❏ ½ cup of onion, cut fine
- ❏ 4 tablespoons of butter or margarine
- ❏ 4 tablespoons of salt
- ❏ ¼ teaspoon of cayenne
- ❏ ½ teaspoon of black pepper
- ❏ 1 teaspoon of celery seed
- ❏ 5 cups of a rich cornbread, crumbled
- ❏ 6 slices of whole wheat bread, toasted slightly
- ❏ ½ cup of minced parsley

1. Grind the gizzard and heart and simmer in a quart of water until tender.

2. Sauté celery, shallots and onion in the butter until done but not brown.

3. Add most of the seasonings.

4. Mix well the cornbread and the toasted whole wheat bread which has been soaked in cold water and squeezed dry.

5. Combine these two mixtures, adding parsley and liver that has been minced, cooked giblets and as much of the liquor from the giblets as is needed to make a moist dressing.

6. Add the rest of the seasonings in amounts suggested to suit individual taste, then stuff turkey.

Note: Allow about eight cups of stuffing for a 10-pound turkey.

– Mrs. V.B. McCutchen
Jennings (Jefferson Davis Parish)

*R*ICE DRESSING

- ❑ 2 tablespoons of flour
- ❑ 2 tablespoons of vegetable oil
- ❑ 1 cup of chopped onions
- ❑ 1 cup of chopped celery
- ❑ ½ cup of chopped bellpepper
- ❑ 2 garlic cloves, minced
- ❑ ½ pound of lean ground beef
- ❑ ½ pound of lean ground pork
- ❑ ½ pound of chicken giblets, chopped
- ❑ 2 teaspoons of salt
- ❑ ¾ teaspoon of black pepper
- ❑ ¾ teaspoon of red pepper
- ❑ 1 cup of chicken broth or water
- ❑ 3 cups of hot cooked rice
- ❑ 1 cup of sliced green onion tops

1. Brown flour in oil until it is a deep red-brown, stirring constantly to prevent burning.

2. Add onion, celery, bellpepper, and garlic; cook until vegetables are tender.

3. Stir-in beef, pork, giblets, and seasonings. Continue cooking until meat loses its color.

4. Blend-in broth; cover and simmer 25 minutes.

5. Stir-in rice and onion tops. Cook five minutes longer. Mixture should be slightly moist.

Makes six servings.

– The Rice Council of America

CORNBREAD DRESSING II

- ❏ 1½ pounds of ground beef
- ❏ Salt, black pepper and red pepper, to taste
- ❏ 1 large onion, chopped
- ❏ ½ cup of chopped bellpepper
- ❏ ¼ cup of chopped celery
- ❏ 1 teaspoon of garlic powder
- ❏ ¼ cup of oil
- ❏ ½ pound of liver, ground
- ❏ 2 cups of water
- ❏ 2 cans of mushroom sauce
- ❏ ½ cup of chopped green onion tops
- ❏ 1 cup of olives, stuffed with pimientos, chopped
- ❏ Cornbread, broken up (Recipe follows)

1. Season ground beef with salt, black pepper and red pepper. Place in heavy pot with onion, bellpepper, celery, garlic and oil; cook until onions and bellpeppers start to brown.

2. Add liver; stir well and cook a few minutes. Add water and mushroom sauce; simmer a few minutes more.

3. Add green onion tops, olives and broken-up Cornbread; mix well. Add extra water or gravy if too dry.

CORNBREAD

- ❏ 2 cups of yellow cornmeal
- ❏ ½ cup of flour
- ❏ 2 eggs
- ❏ 2 teaspoons of baking powder
- ❏ 1 teaspoon of sugar
- ❏ 1¼ cups of buttermilk
- ❏ 1 teaspoon of salt

1. Mix all ingredients in a mixing bowl.

2. Pour into a greased pan and bake at 425 degrees for 25 to 30 minutes.

3. Remove from pan and cool before breaking up and adding to dressing.

– Mrs. Jessie Hoffpauir
Indian Bayou (Vermilion Parish)

OYSTER & RICE DRESSING

- ❏ 1 pint of chicken liver
- ❏ 1 pint of chicken gizzards
- ❏ ¼ cup of oil
- ❏ 1 onion, chopped
- ❏ 2 bellpeppers, chopped
- ❏ ½ stalk of celery, chopped
- ❏ 6 cups of cooked rice
- ❏ Salt, black pepper and cayenne pepper, to taste
- ❏ 1 pint of fresh oysters, chopped

1. Boil liver and gizzards in water to cover until tender, about 30 minutes; save broth and grind liver and gizzards in food processor or grinder.

2. In oil, sauté onion, bellpepper and celery until onions are transparent; add ground liver and gizzards; simmer for 15 minutes; then add cooked rice and enough broth to make dressing moist.

3. Season dressing with salt, black pepper and cayenne pepper; add oysters and mix well.

4. Dressing may be used to stuff a turkey or hen, or it may be placed in a buttered casserole dish and baked at 325 degrees for 45 minutes.

Makes eight servings.

*E*GGPLANT *D*RESSING

- 3 large eggplants, peeled and cubed
- 1 large onion, chopped
- 2 tablespoons of shortening
- 1 link of smoked sausage, ground
- Salt and pepper, to taste
- 3 cups of cooked rice or cornbread

1. Place eggplant in cool salt water to prevent discoloration.

2. Sauté onion in shortening; add ground sausage. Cook together for five minutes.

3. Add drained eggplant, salt and pepper. Cook about 10 minutes or until eggplant becomes soft and tender.

4. Mix with rice or cornbread.

Note: Do not use an iron pot for this recipe.

– Lammie Normand
Marksville (Avoyelles Parish)

*E*GGPLANT & *B*EEF *C*ASSEROLE

- ❏ 2 tablespoons of butter
- ❏ 2 medium onions, chopped
- ❏ 1 garlic clove, minced
- ❏ 1½ pounds of ground beef
- ❏ 1 tablespoon of tomato paste
- ❏ 3 tablespoons of chopped parsley
- ❏ ½ cup of dry white wine
- ❏ Salt and pepper, to taste
- ❏ 3 large eggplants, sliced 1/2-inch thick but not peeled
- ❏ 4 tablespoons of olive oil
- ❏ 1 egg, beaten
- ❏ Breadcrumbs
- ❏ Grated Parmesan cheese
- ❏ Butter
- ❏ Cream Sauce (Recipe follows)

1. Sauté onions and garlic in butter. Add ground beef and sauté until onions and beef are browned.

2. Add tomato paste, parsley, wine and seasonings to taste. Cover skillet and simmer slowly until meat is well-cooked and the juices have almost been absorbed.

3. Fry eggplant in olive oil in another skillet until golden brown.

4. Add beaten egg to meat mixture along with three tablespoons of breadcrumbs. Mix well.

5. Sprinkle the bottom of a buttered casserole with breadcrumbs. Place one-third of the eggplant over crumbs. Top with one-half of the meat mixture, and liberally sprinkle meat with grated Parmesan cheese. Place another third of the eggplant, remaining meat, more cheese and then top with the remaining third of the eggplant.

6. Pour Cream Sauce over the entire casserole; sprinkle with more Parmesan cheese and breadcrumbs. Dot with butter.

7. Bake uncovered at 350 degrees for 45 minutes or until golden brown.

CREAM SAUCE

- ❑ 1¾ cups of milk
- ❑ 3 tablespoons of melted butter
- ❑ 1 egg yolk
- ❑ ¼ cup of sherry
- ❑ 2 tablespoons of flour
- ❑ Salt and pepper, to taste
- ❑ Pinch of nutmeg

1. Bring milk to a boil; add melted butter, egg yolk and sherry.

2. Thicken with the flour and season with salt, pepper and nutmeg, stirring constantly to keep mixture smooth.

– John R. Thistlethwaite
Opelousas (St. Landry Parish)

Sweet Potato Casserole

- 3 cups of cooked and mashed fresh sweet potatoes
- ¾ stick of butter, melted
- 1 cup of evaporated milk
- 2 eggs, beaten
- ½ teaspoon of nutmeg
- ½ teaspoon of cinnamon
- 1 teaspoon of vanilla
- Topping (Recipe follows)

1. Combine first seven ingredients; pour into baking dish.

2. Top with Topping.

3. Bake uncovered at 425 degrees for 15 minutes.

TOPPING

- 1 cup of crushed corn flakes
- ½ cup of chopped nuts
- ½ cup of brown sugar
- ¾ stick of butter, melted

Combine all four ingredients.

– Doris D. Jacob
Reserve (St. John the Baptist Parish)

Breads & Cereals

The most famous scene in Grand Coteau, La., includes a crucifix framed by ancient moss-draped oaks and overlooking an old Jesuit cemetery behind Our Lady of the Oaks Retreat House. The town is known as a center for religious retreats and Catholic education.

COUCHE COUCHE

- ❑ ¼ cup of oil
- ❑ 2 cups of cornmeal
- ❑ 1½ teaspoons of salt
- ❑ 1 teaspoon of baking powder
- ❑ ¾ cup of milk
- ❑ ¾ cup of water

1. Using a heavy iron pot, heat the oil.

2. Mix dry ingredients; add milk and water. (Batter will be soft.)

3. Pour batter in hot oil; let crust form on bottom before stirring. Put on low heat and stir occasionally, until *couche couche* is cooked, about 15 minutes.

4. Serve in bowl with milk and sugar, as a cereal.

– Mrs. Ralph Gonsoulin
New Iberia (Iberia Parish)

*P*AIN *P*ERDU
*(L*OST *B*READ*)*

- ❑ 3 eggs
- ❑ ¼ cup of sugar
- ❑ ½ teaspoon of salt
- ❑ 2 cups of milk
- ❑ 12 slices of bread

1. Beat eggs, sugar and salt; add milk.

2. Dip slices of bread into mixture and fry in slight amount of hot fat until delicate brown on both sides.

3. Serve hot; sprinkle with powdered sugar or serve with syrup.

– Dot Robert
Iberville Parish

𝓕RENCH DOUGHNUTS

- ❑ 1 cup of boiling water
- ❑ ¼ cup of shortening
- ❑ ½ cup of sugar
- ❑ 1 teaspoon of salt
- ❑ 1 cup of evaporated milk
- ❑ 1 cake of yeast, softened in 1/2 cup of lukewarm water
- ❑ 2 eggs, well-beaten
- ❑ 7½ cups of sifted flour

1. Pour boiling water over shortening, sugar and salt.

2. Add milk.

3. When lukewarm, add yeast that has been softened in water.

4. Add beaten eggs.

5. Stir-in four cups of flour and beat hard.

6. Add enough flour to make a soft dough.

7. Place in a greased bowl.

8. Grease top of dough. Cover with waxed paper and a lid, or cloth, and keep in the refrigerator until ready to use.

9. Roll dough to one-fourth-inch thickness. Cut with scalloped cookie cutter. (Do not let dough rise before frying.)

10. Fry in hot deep fat (360 degrees); brown one side, turn, and brown on the other. Drain on absorbent paper.

11. Cover with a thin frosting.

Makes 60 doughnuts.

FRENCH BREAD

- ❏ 2¼ cups of warm water (110 degrees)
- ❏ 1 envelope of dry yeast
- ❏ 1 teaspoon of sugar
- ❏ 7 to 8 cups of sifted flour
- ❏ Salt
- ❏ 1 tablespoon of butter, softened
- ❏ ½ cup of cornmeal

1. Combine one-fourth cup of warm water with yeast and sugar and let mixture set for 10 minutes or until mixture doubles in bulk.

2. Add yeast mixture to seven cups of flour, one tablespoon of salt and the remaining two cups of warm water; mix well until the dough can be gathered into a ball.

3. Knead dough, adding more flour if necessary (up to one cup) until dough is no longer sticky.

4. Spread butter on the inside of a large bowl and place dough in bowl, turning dough until surface is coated with butter; cover and let dough stand in a warm place until it doubles in bulk.

5. Punch the dough down and divide into three pieces; shape each piece into a loaf about two inches in diameter and 15 inches long and place on a cookie sheet dusted with cornmeal. Cut five or six diagonal slashes across the top of each loaf.

6. Mix half a teaspoon of salt with half a cup of water; brush each loaf with this mixture, cover and let rise until double in bulk.

7. Place large, shallow baking pan half filled with water on the bottom of the oven; bake loaves at 400 degrees for 15 minutes.

8. Lower heat to 350 degrees, brush bread with water-salt mixture and continue to bake for 30 minutes (basting again with water-salt mixture) until loaves are golden brown; cool on a wire rack.

*S*WEET *P*OTATO *B*READ *& M*UFFINS

- ½ cup of butter or oleo
- ½ cup of shortening
- 2½ cups of sugar
- 4 eggs
- 2 cups of cold, mashed sweet potatoes
- 3½ cups of sifted flour
- 1 teaspoon of salt
- 1 teaspoon of ground cinnamon
- 1½ teaspoons of ground nutmeg
- 2 teaspoons of baking soda
- 1 cup of chopped walnuts
- ¾ cup of cold, strong, dark coffee

1. Cream butter, shortening and sugar; add eggs, one at a time, mixing well after each addition.

2. Blend-in sweet potatoes.

3. Sift together dry ingredients; add nuts.

4. Stir into creamed mixture alternately with cold coffee.

5. Pour batter into two greased 9 x 5 x 3 loaf pans and eight greased muffin pan cups.

6. Bake at 375 degrees for one hour for loaves and 25 minutes for muffins or until they test done in the center.

7. Cool 10 minutes, remove from pans, and cool completely.

– Mrs. Charles F. Hebert
Cameron (Cameron Parish)

Jeanerette Sugar Co. is among the dozen or so mills that grind cane and make sugar and molasses in the fall in south Louisiana. The sugarcane industry has been a part of the fabric of life in this region for many generations.

OLD-FASHIONED SYRUP CAKE

- ❑ ½ cup of sugar
- ❑ ½ cup of butter or oleo
- ❑ 2 cups of syrup
- ❑ 2 eggs
- ❑ 2 cups of flour
- ❑ 1 teaspoon of salt
- ❑ ½ teaspoon of soda
- ❑ ½ cup of buttermilk
- ❑ 2 teaspoons of vanilla

1. Mix sugar, butter and syrup together; add eggs and mix well.

2. Add flour, salt and soda, alternating with buttermilk; add vanilla.

3. Bake in a greased and floured tube pan at 350 degrees for 45 minutes to one hour.

– Jeanette M. Guidry
Breaux Bridge (St. Martin Parish)

Molasses Candy

- ❑ 2 cups of molasses
- ❑ 1 tablespoon of sugar
- ❑ 1/4 cup of butter
- ❑ 1/3 teaspoon of soda

1. Cook molasses and one tablespoon of sugar, stirring occasionally while boiling.

2. Stir-in butter and soda.

3. Pour into buttered tins. Pull when cool.

– Mrs. H.E. Demmon
Jennings (Jefferson Davis Parish)

OREILLES DE COCHON
(PIG'S EARS)

- ☐ 1¾ cups of all-purpose flour
- ☐ 2 teaspoons of baking powder
- ☐ ½ teaspoon of salt
- ☐ 2 eggs
- ☐ 6 tablespoons of butter or oleo, melted and cooled
- ☐ Oil for deep-fat frying
- ☐ ¾ cup of cane syrup
- ☐ ½ cup of chopped pecans

1. Stir together flour, baking powder and salt; set aside.

2. In mixer bowl, beat eggs until frothy; gradually add cooled butter, beating constantly. Beat-in two-thirds of the dry ingredients, a little at a time. By hand, stir-in remaining dry ingredients.

3. Divide dough into 24 portions; shape each piece of dough into a ball. On lightly floured surface, roll out each ball to a thin circle, about five inches in diameter.

4. Fry dough rounds one or two at a time in deep hot fat (375 degrees). As rounds rise to surface of oil, insert one tine of long-tined fork through the center, twisting slightly to fold and curl edges (forming pig's ears). Fry until golden brown, about two minutes, turning once. Drain fried pastry on paper towels.

5. In a small saucepan, combine syrup and pecans; heat just to simmering. Drizzle warm syrup-pecan mixture over pastries.

Makes 24 pastries.

– Mrs. Sam Broussard
New Iberia (Iberia Parish)

𝒴AM-PECAN CAKE

- ❑ 1 box of orange gelatin
- ❑ 1/2 cup of boiling water
- ❑ 1 box of yellow cake mix
- ❑ 1 cup of chopped pecans
- ❑ 4 eggs
- ❑ 2/3 cup of salad oil
- ❑ 1 cup of mashed yams
- ❑ 1/4 cup of orange juice
- ❑ 1 teaspoon of grated orange rind

1. Dissolve gelatin in boiling water.

2. Place cake mix in bowl; add pecans and mix well.

3. Add dissolved gelatin, eggs, salad oil, yams, orange juice and rind to cake mix; mix according to directions on cake mix box.

4. Pour into greased bundt pan; bake at 350 degrees for one hour. Can be glazed if desired.

– Janet Matte
Breaux Bridge (St. Martin Parish)

*P*RALINE COOKIES

- ❑ 1 cup of light brown sugar
- ❑ 1 tablespoon of flour
- ❑ 1/3 teaspoon of salt
- ❑ 1 egg white, beaten
- ❑ 1 teaspoon of vanilla
- ❑ 2 cups of pecans

1. Mix sugar, flour and salt; sift.

2. Add beaten egg white, vanilla and pecans.

3. Drop by the teaspoonful on cookie sheet heavily greased with shortening.

4. Bake at 275 degrees for 35 minutes. Remove from cookie sheet before cookies are cold.

– Mrs. A.A. Smith
New Roads (Pointe Coupee Parish)

$\mathcal{L}$OUISIANA FIG CAKE

- ❑ 1 large egg
- ❑ 2 tablespoons of sugar
- ❑ 1 teaspoon of vanilla
- ❑ ½ cup of salad oil
- ❑ 1¼ cups of flour
- ❑ ½ teaspoon of baking powder
- ❑ ½ teaspoon of salt
- ❑ 1 pint of fig preserves

1. Grease and flour a 9 x 9 x 2-inch pan; preheat oven to 350 degrees.

2. Place the egg, sugar and vanilla in a mixing bowl and beat slightly with a spoon; add the salad oil and beat again.

3. Sift the dry ingredients all at once and add them to the above mixture; add the fig preserves to this batter and stir.

4. Pour batter into the prepared pan, smooth, and bake for 35 to 40 minutes.

– Mrs. Meredith Hebert
New Iberia (Iberia Parish)

CHRISTMAS CAKE

- ☐ ½ pound of butter
- ☐ ½ pound of oleo
- ☐ 3½ cups of light brown sugar
- ☐ 6 eggs
- ☐ 4 cups of plain flour
- ☐ 1 teaspoon of baking powder
- ☐ 1 pound of raisins
- ☐ 3 cups of nuts (walnuts and pecans)
- ☐ ½ cup of brandy (peach or apricot)

1. Mix ingredients in the order given in a very large bowl.

2. Pour batter into a well-greased and -floured tube pan.

3. Bake at 350 degrees for two hours or more.

– Cookie Hutcherson
Houma (Terrebonne Parish)

$\mathcal{L}$OUISIANA PEAR CAKE

- ❑ 1 stick of margarine, softened
- ❑ 1 cup of sugar
- ❑ 1 egg
- ❑ 1½ cups of flour
- ❑ ¼ teaspoon of salt
- ❑ 1 teaspoon of soda
- ❑ ½ teaspoon of cinnamon
- ❑ 1 teaspoon of vanilla
- ❑ 2 cups of grated raw pears
- ❑ ½ cup of chopped pecans

1. Mix margarine, sugar and egg together.

2. Sift flour, salt, soda and cinnamon together; add to sugar and egg mixture.

3. Add vanilla, pears and nuts.

4. Pour into a greased and floured baking pan 8 x 8 x 2 inches.

5. Bake at 300 degrees for one hour; serve with whipped cream or Cool Whip.

– Mercedes Lormand
Hathaway (Jefferson Davis Parish)

$\mathcal{F}$IG COFFEECAKE

- ❑ 2 eggs, beaten
- ❑ 3/4 cup of sugar
- ❑ 1/3 cup of butter, melted
- ❑ 1½ cups of flour
- ❑ 1½ teaspoons of baking powder
- ❑ 1/2 teaspoon of salt
- ❑ 1/2 cup of milk
- ❑ 1 teaspoon of vanilla
- ❑ Fig Mixture (Recipe follows)

1. Combine eggs, sugar and butter; beat well.

2. In a separate bowl, combine flour, baking powder and salt.

3. Gradually add flour mixture to egg mixture alternately with milk.

4. Stir-in vanilla.

5. Pour one-half of the batter into a greased and floured eight-inch-square pan; top with one-half of the Fig Mixture. Pour remaining batter over fig layer, then top with remaining Fig Mixture.

6. Bake at 350 degrees for 40 to 45 minutes or until cake tests done.

FIG MIXTURE

- ❑ 1/2 cup of packed brown sugar
- ❑ 2 tablespoons of softened butter
- ❑ 1/2 teaspoon of ground cinnamon
- ❑ 10 fig bars, crumbled

Combine all ingredients; mix well.

– LSU Cooperative Extension Service
Lafayette Parish

*P*ECAN *P*RALINES 1

- ❏ 4 cups of sugar, divided
- ❏ 1 teaspoon of salt
- ❏ 2 cups of cream (or one large can of evaporated milk)
- ❏ 3 cups of pecans

1. In a heavy pot, make a syrup with three cups of sugar, salt and cream. Cook for about eight minutes.

2. In another heavy pot or heavy skillet, melt one cup of sugar slowly over very low heat, constantly stirring until caramelized.

3. Pour caramelized sugar into the boiling syrup at one time, stirring constantly and rapidly.

4. Boil this mixture (without stirring) to a temperature of 238 degrees, or to a soft-ball stage (about two minutes).

5. Pour into a flat pan or crock. Beat until it begins to be creamy; add the nuts.

6. Drop by the spoonful onto waxed paper to form flat, round cakes.

– Blanche Arceneaux Swann
Marksville (Avoyelles Parish)

CAJUN CAKE

- ❑ 2 cups of flour
- ❑ 1½ cups of sugar
- ❑ 2 teaspoons of baking soda
- ❑ 2 small cans of crushed pineapple, with juice
- ❑ 2 eggs
- ❑ Icing (Recipe follows)

1. Mix all ingredients well.

2. Bake in a square pan for 30 minutes at 350 degrees.

3. Cool and ice cake.

ICING

- ❑ ½ can of evaporated milk
- ❑ ¼ pound of butter or oleo
- ❑ ¾ cup of sugar
- ❑ 1 package of coconut
- ❑ ½ cup of chopped pecans

Cook evaporated milk, butter and sugar until very thick. Add coconut and pecans.

– Thelma Smith
Rayne (Acadia Parish)

PECAN PRALINES II

- ❑ 2 2/3 cups of sugar
- ❑ 1 cup of evaporated milk
- ❑ 1/2 cup of butter
- ❑ 2 tablespoons of white corn syrup
- ❑ 2 cups of pecan halves
- ❑ 1 teaspoon of vanilla extract

1. In a two-quart heavy saucepan, mix sugar, evaporated milk, butter and corn syrup.

2. Cook until a teaspoonful of the mixture forms a soft ball (235 degrees) when dropped in water.

3. Remove from heat and add pecans and vanilla extract.

4. Beat until very thick and heavy.

5. Drop by the teaspoonful onto waxed paper placed on cloth. (This makes pralines easier to pick up.)

Makes 30 pralines.

– Mae St. Marie
Houma (Terrebonne Parish)

Fig Bar

- ❑ 4 eggs
- ❑ 2 cups of sugar
- ❑ 1 cup of melted margarine
- ❑ 1 teaspoon of salt
- ❑ 1 teaspoon of baking powder
- ❑ 2 cups of flour
- ❑ 1 teaspoon of almond flavoring
- ❑ 1 teaspoon of lemon flavoring
- ❑ 2 cups of chopped, drained fig preserves
- ❑ 1 cup of chopped nuts

1. Beat eggs well; gradually add sugar and margarine.

2. Add dry ingredients and flavorings; beat well.

3. Fold-in figs and nuts.

4. Pour into well-greased and -floured jelly roll pan, 15½ x 10½ inches.

5. Bake at 350 degrees for 30 minutes.

6. Cut into bars immediately after baking.

– Mrs. Don A. Marx
Crowley (Acadia Parish)

TARTE A LA BOUILLIE
(CREAM CUSTARD PIE)

- ❑ ½ cup of sugar
- ❑ 3 tablespoons of flour
- ❑ 2 eggs
- ❑ 2½ cups of milk
- ❑ 2 teaspoons of vanilla
- ❑ Sweet Dough Pie Shell (Recipe follows)

1. Mix sugar and flour together; add beaten eggs.

2. Bring milk to a boil; add a small amount of hot milk to egg mixture, stirring well. Add this to remaining hot milk and cook until thick.

3. Add vanilla and cool slightly.

4. Pour into prepared Sweet Dough Pie Shell and cover top of custard with little strips of the dough.

5. Bake at 400 degrees for 30 to 35 minutes.

SWEET DOUGH PIE SHELL

- ☐ ½ cup of sugar (less, if desired)
- ☐ ¼ pound of butter or oil
- ☐ 1 egg, beaten
- ☐ 2 teaspoons of vanilla
- ☐ 3 cups of flour
- ☐ 2 teaspoons of baking powder
- ☐ ½ cup of milk
- ☐ ½ teaspoon of salt

1. Cream sugar and butter; add egg and vanilla, mixing well.

2. Alternately add flour, baking powder and milk with salt.

3. Roll out dough and place in pie plate, saving a small amount of dough for strips over the pie.

– Mrs. Lillian Schifani
Thibodaux (Lafourche Parish)

Sweet Potato Pie

- ❑ 1 cup of mashed cooked sweet potatoes
- ❑ ¼ pound of butter, melted
- ❑ 1½ cups of sugar
- ❑ 3 tablespoons of flour
- ❑ 2 eggs
- ❑ 1 small can of evaporated milk
- ❑ 1 teaspoon of lemon extract
- ❑ 1 teaspoon of vanilla
- ❑ 1 unbaked pie crust

1. Mix first eight ingredients together.

2. Pour in unbaked nine-inch pie shell.

3. Bake one hour at 350 degrees. Serve warm.

– Mrs. Hadley Fontenot
Jennings (Jefferson Davis Parish)

FRENCH EGG CUSTARD

- ❑ 3 cups of whole milk
- ❑ 15 eggs
- ❑ 2½ cups of sugar or honey
- ❑ 1½ cans of evaporated milk (13-ounce cans)
- ❑ ½ cup of vanilla extract

1. Heat whole milk until just before boiling point.

2. In a large mixing bowl, combine eggs and sugar and beat with whisk until frothy.

3. Add evaporated milk and vanilla to egg mixture and mix well.

4. Gradually beat-in heated milk.

5. Pour into pan 15 x 11 x 2 inches. Bake at 350 degrees until firm and lightly brown.

6. Let cool to room temperature and serve in sherbet glasses.

– Randolph's Restaurant
Golden Meadow (Lafourche Parish)

*P*ECAN PIE

- ❑ 1 cup of brown sugar
- ❑ ½ cup of white sugar
- ❑ 1 tablespoon of flour
- ❑ 2 eggs
- ❑ 2 tablespoons of milk
- ❑ 1 teaspoon of vanilla
- ❑ ¼ pound of butter, melted
- ❑ 1 cup of chopped pecans
- ❑ Unbaked pie shell

1. Combine first eight ingredients.

2. Pour in unbaked pie shell.

3. Bake at 375 degrees for 40 minutes.

– Mrs. Goldie B. Lowe
Port Allen (West Baton Rouge Parish)

OLD-FASHIONED BREAD PUDDING

- ❑ 4 cups of milk
- ❑ 8 slices of stale bread
- ❑ 4 eggs, separated
- ❑ 1½ cups of sugar
- ❑ 1 small can of evaporated milk
- ❑ 1 teaspoon of vanilla
- ❑ 1 cup of coconut (optional)
- ❑ 4 tablespoons of sugar

1. Heat milk, pour over bread and mash.

2. Cream egg yolks and sugar; add to bread mixture. Add evaporated milk, vanilla and coconut; mix well.

3. Bake uncovered in buttered pan at 375 degrees for one hour.

4. Beat egg whites with four tablespoons of sugar until stiff and sugar is dissolved. Spoon over pudding.

5. Return to oven and brown the top at 350 degrees.

– Mrs. Ralph Gonsoulin
New Iberia (Iberia Parish)

*P*ECAN TASSIES

- ❏ 2 tablespoons of butter or oleo, creamed
- ❏ 1 cup of brown sugar
- ❏ 2 eggs
- ❏ 1 cup of ground pecans
- ❏ 2 tablespoons of vanilla
- ❏ Shells (Recipe follows)

1. Combine butter, sugar, and eggs; add pecans and vanilla; blend well.

2. Fill each Shell with pecan filling (about three-fourths full).

3. Bake at 325 degrees for 25 minutes.

4. Cool in tins for about five minutes before removing.

Makes about three dozen little pecan pies.

SHELLS

- ❏ ¼ pound of oleo or butter
- ❏ 1 3-ounce package of cream cheese
- ❏ 1 cup of sifted flour
- ❏ Pinch of salt

1. Cream oleo and cream cheese until well blended. Add flour and salt; mix well. Let stand for one hour.

2. Take small balls of dough and work well with thumb into miniature muffin tins to form thin shells.

– Shirley Miller
Plaquemine (Iberville Parish)

BLACKBERRY DUMPLINGS

- ❑ 4 tablespoons of butter
- ❑ 1 cup of milk
- ❑ 2 eggs
- ❑ 3½ cups of sugar, divided
- ❑ 2 teaspoons of vanilla
- ❑ 3½ cups of flour
- ❑ 3 teaspoons of baking powder
- ❑ 4 cups of water
- ❑ 1½ quarts of blackberries

1. Melt butter and allow to cool; mix with the milk, eggs, one cup of the sugar and vanilla; add dry ingredients. Do not overmix.

2. Combine four cups of water, two and a half cups of sugar and blackberries; cook over medium heat until mixture thickens.

3. Drop dough by the spoonful or in little balls into blackberry mixture and cook until dough rises.

4. Test with fork; when it comes out clean, remove the dumpling and continue adding dumplings until all dough is used.

Serve warm with blackberry mixture.

Makes three to four dozen.

– Mrs. Gayle Boudreaux
Terrebonne Parish

RICE PUDDING

- ❑ 2 eggs
- ❑ 2 cups of milk
- ❑ 1¼ cups of cold, cooked rice
- ❑ 1 cup of seedless raisins
- ❑ ½ cup of sugar
- ❑ ¼ teaspoon of salt
- ❑ 1 teaspoon of vanilla extract
- ❑ Dash of ground cinnamon and nutmeg

1. Beat eggs until light and thick; add milk.

2. Lightly mix in the other ingredients; place in a buttered one and one-half quart casserole.

3. Bake in a shallow pan of water at 350 degrees for one hour, or until mixture is firm.

Makes six servings.

– Mrs. Mildredge Broussard
Grand Chenier (Cameron Parish)

"Tac-Tac"
(Popcorn Balls)

- 1/2 cup of sugar
- 2/3 cup of sugarcane syrup
- 1/3 cup of water
- 1 teaspoon of vinegar
- 1/4 teaspoon of salt
- 1 tablespoon of butter
- 1/8 teaspoon of soda
- 4 cups of popped popcorn
- 2 cups of shelled peanuts

1. Combine sugar, syrup, water, vinegar and salt. Stir until sugar dissolves.

2. Cook over a medium flame to light crack stage.

3. Remove from heat and add butter and soda.

4. Stir well and pour over popped corn and peanuts.

5. Butter your hands and form the mixture into balls.

Index

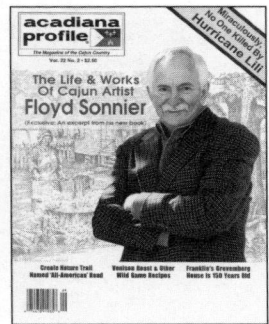

Everything you always wanted to know about the Cajun Country of South Louisiana can be found in the pages of **Acadiana Profile.**

Price: The magazine is published six times a year. The rates are: 6 issues for $21, 12 issues for $40, 18 issues for $59, and 24 issues for $78.

To Subscribe: Either call in your order to (800) 850-8851, or mail it in to Acadiana Profile, P.O. Box 52247, Lafayette, LA 70505. You may pay with check, money order or credit card (VISA, MC, or AmEx). Be sure to include your name and mailing address and the number of issues for which you'd like to subscribe.

Regional Books
About
Intriguing

South Louisiana

(Please turn the page)

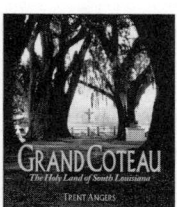

Grand Coteau
The Holy Land of South Louisiana

A 176-page hardcover book that captures the spirit of one of the truly holy places in North America. It is a town of mystery, with well-established ties to the supernatural, including the famous Miracle of Grand Coteau. Brought to life by dozens of exceptional color photographs, the book focuses on the town's major religious institutions: The Academy of the Sacred Heart, Our Lady of the Oaks Retreat House and St. Charles College/Jesuit Spirituality Center. The book explores not only the history of these three institutions but also the substance of their teachings. (Author: Trent Angers. ISBN: 0-925417-47-5. Price: $44.95)

The Truth About The Cajuns

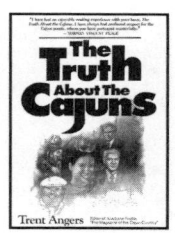

A 120-page paperback book that describes the French-Acadian, or Cajun, people with the accuracy and dignity to which they are entitled – contrary to the shallow, stereotyping manner in which they have been depicted by many of the news media. This controversial book sets the record straight about the Cajun people and their culture. Illustrated with maps and photos. (Author: Trent Angers. ISBN: 0-925417-29-7. Price: $11.95)

Louisiana's French Heritage

A 192-page hardcover book about the French contribution to the colonization of the New World. It describes the settlement of the Acadian Peninsula, the discovery and exploration of the Mississippi River, the development of the first Louisiana colony and the exile of the French-Acadians from Canada. Illustrated with maps and historical drawings. (Author: Truman Stacey. ISBN: 0-925417-02-5. Price: $15.95)

From Small Bits of Charcoal
The Life & Works Of A Cajun Artist

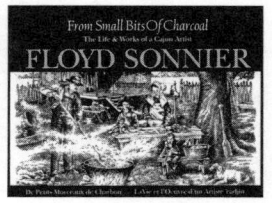

This 190-page hardcover book is the autobiography of pen-and-ink artist Floyd Sonnier (1933-2002) of Lafayette, La. Written and illustrated by Mr. Sonnier, the book tells the story of growing up as a French-speaking Cajun in rural south Louisiana in the 1940s and '50s. It is also a testament to his love of his French-Acadian, or Cajun, culture and heritage. (ISBN: 0-925417-46-7. Price: $59.95)

Dudley LeBlanc: A Biography

A 104-page softcover book about Dudley LeBlanc, the most famous Cajun of all time, and unquestionably one of Louisiana's most unforgettable characters. The political leader of the Cajun people in the 1930s, '40s, '50s and '60s, "Coozan Dud" also invented and promoted HADACOL into the best-selling patent medicine in America in its time. (Author: Trent Angers. ISBN: 0-925417-12-2. Price: $9.95)

Dreaming Impossible Dreams
Reflections of an Entrepreneur

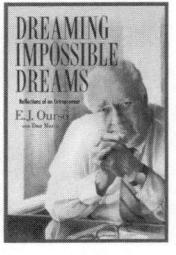

This 176-page autobiography is the rags-to-riches story of multimillionaire philanthropist E.J. Ourso of Donaldsonville, Louisiana, the man for whom the LSU Business School is named. It reveals how Ourso acquired 56 businesses in 48 years – the first 25 with no money down. A testament to the effectiveness of the American free enterprise system, the book chronicles Ourso's life beginning with his early years as a salesman. It reveals his secrets to the acquisition of wealth. (Author: E.J. Ourso with Dan Marin. Hardcover ISBN: 0-925417-42-4, Price: $22.95; Softcover ISBN: 0-925417-43-2, Price: $14.95)

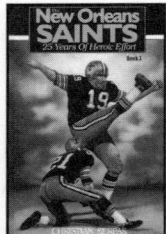

The New Orleans Saints
25 Years of Heroic Effort

A set of 2 hardcover books (112 and 184 pages) describes the colorful history of the Saints from 1967 thru 1991, featuring Tom Dempsey, Archie Manning, Bobby Hebert, Dalton Hilliard, Morten Andersen, "The Dome Patrol" and many more. Illustrated with photos. (ISBN: 0-925417-09-2 and 0-925417-11-4. Price: $25 for the set)

The Top 100 CAJUN Recipes Of All Time

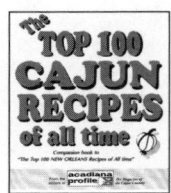

A 160-page hardcover book containing 100 recipes selected by the editors of *Acadiana Profile*, "The Magazine of the Cajun Country." For example, Boudin, Couche Couche, Maque Choux, Mirliton, Crawfish Etouffee, Chicken Fricassee, Pralines–the classics of South Louisiana cuisine. (Hardcover ISBN: 0-925417-52-1, Price $14.95; Softcover, 7x10 size with 48 pages, ISBN: 0-925417-20-3, Price: $7.95)

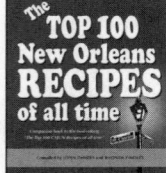

The Top 100 NEW ORLEANS Recipes Of All Time

A 192-page hardcover book containing 100 of the recipes that have helped to make New Orleans food world-famous. For example, Shrimp Creole, Red Beans & Rice, Blackened Redfish, Oyster Loaf, Muffaletta, Beignets, Café au Lait and King Cake. (ISBN: 0-925417-51-3. Price: $14.95)

Cajun Cooking For Beginners

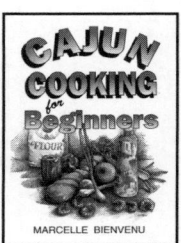

A 48-page saddle-stitched soft cover book that teaches the basics of authentic Cajun cooking. It contains about 50 simple, easy-to-follow recipes; cooking tips and hints; a glossary of Cajun food terms, such as roux, gumbo, jambalaya and etouffee; and definitions of basic cooking terms, such as beat, blend, broil, sauté and simmer. (Author: Marcelle Bienvenu. ISBN: 0-925417-23-8. Price: $7.95)

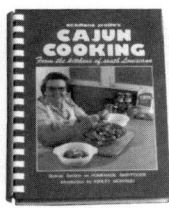

Cajun Cooking, Part 1...

...contains about 400 of the best Cajun recipes, like Jambalaya, Crawfish Pie, Filé Gumbo, Cochon de Lait, Chicken & Okra Gumbo, Sauce Piquante. Special features include a section on homemade baby foods and drawings of classic south Louisiana scenery. (ISBN: 0-925417-38-6. Price: $17.95)

Cajun Cooking, Part 2...

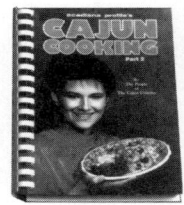

...picks up where Part 1 left off. It contains such delicious dishes as Shrimp & Crab Bisque, Fresh Vegetable Soup, Seafood-Stuffed Bellpepper, Broiled Seafood Platter, Yam-Pecan Cake. The recipes appear in the same easy-to-follow format as in Part 1, except they're in real large print for an arm's-length reading. (ISBN: 0-925417-05-X. Price: $15.95)

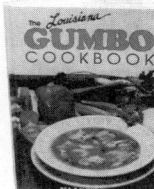

The Louisiana GUMBO Cookbook

A 192-page hardcover book with more than 100 recipes for the Cajun and Creole gumbo dishes that have made south Louisiana food world-famous. Special sections on the history of gumbo and filé, plus instructions for making rice and gumbo stocks. (Authors: Bea & Floyd Weber. ISBN: 0-925417-13-0. Price: $17.95)

Nicky The Swamp Dog
A *True Story*

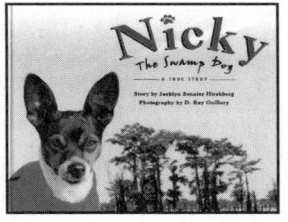

A 40-page hardcover book about an intriguing little dog that lives in the Atchafalaya Basin in south Louisiana. She and her master ("Half Pint" Guillory) rescue lost and injured animals – such as nutria, beavers and owls – and bring them back to their houseboat. Here, they feed them, shelter them and nurse them back to health. Then, when they are well, they release them back into the wilds. Lavishly illustrated with photographs of Nicky, her furry and feathered friends, and the swamp environment in which they live. (ISBN: 0-925417-36-X. Price: $14.95)

The Legend of Catfish & Little Bream

A 40-page hardcover book about a big fish who gets bored with life in a little pond in the South. He sets out on a great adventure to the North, and along the way learns some of life's most important lessons – that friendship is priceless, that home is where the heart is, and that the grass isn't always greener on the other side of the hill. Magnificently illustrated! (Author & Illustrator: Ronnie Wells. ISBN: 0-925417-37-8. Price: $19.95)

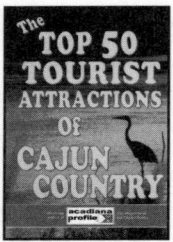

The Top 50 Tourist Attractions Of Cajun Country

A 96-page hardcover book with brief write-ups on the most popular and/or intriguing tourist attractions in south Louisiana, with photos of each, plus an easy-to-follow location map. (ISBN: 0-925417-45-9. Price: $12.95)

The Top 50 Festivals Of Cajun Country

A 48-page saddle-stitched soft cover book with brief write-ups on the biggest and/or most intriguing fairs and festivals in south Louisiana, with beautiful color photos of some. Also, a special section on Mardi Gras, its history, its pageantry, its mystique. (ISBN: 0-925417-32-7. Price: $6.95)

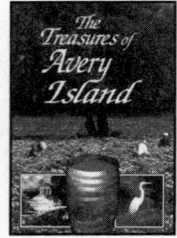

The Treasures of Avery Island

A 24-page softcover book filled with beautiful color pictures and information on exotic Jungle Gardens and the world-renowned TABASCO® Pepper Sauce operation. Alligators and azaleas, bayous and bamboo, as well as great flocks of snowy white egrets, fields of hot peppers, and a gold-layered replica of Buddha are some of the treasures found in this book. (Author: Diane Moore. ISBN: 0-925417-39-4. Price: $4.95)

TO ORDER, list the books you wish to purchase along with the corresponding cost of each. Add shipping & handling cost of $3.00 for the first book and 75¢ per book thereafter. Louisiana residents add 8% tax to the cost of the books. Mail your order and check or credit card authorization (VISA/MC/AmEx) to: Acadian House Publishing, Dept. CHD, P.O. Box 52247, Lafayette, LA 70505. Or call (800) 850-8851.
